DOPPLER ULTRASOUND

Principles and Instruments

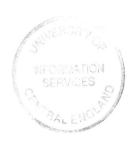

FREDERICK W. KREMKAU, Ph.D.

Professor and Director
Center for Medical Ultrasound
Bowman Gray School of Medicine
Wake Forest University
Winston-Salem, North Carolina

DOPPLER ULTRASOUND

Principles and Instruments

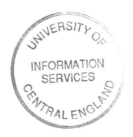

1990

W.B. SAUNDERS COMPANY
Harcourt Brace Jovanovich, Inc.
Philadelphia   London   Toronto
Montreal   Sydney   Tokyo

W. B. SAUNDERS COMPANY
Harcourt Brace Jovanovich, Inc.

The Curtis Center
Independence Square West
Philadelphia, PA 19106

Library of Congress Cataloging-in-Publication Data
Kremkau, Frederick W. Doppler ultrasound : principles and instruments / Frederick W. Kremkau.   p. cm. Includes bibliographical references. ISBN 0-7216-2864-8 1. Doppler ultrasonography. I. Title. [DNLM: 1. Ultrasonic Diagnosis—instrumentation. 2. Ultrasonic Diagnosis—methods. WB 289 K92da] RC78.7.U4K747   1990 616.07′543—dc20 DNLM/DLC <div align="right">90-8134</div>

Editor: W. B. Saunders Staff
Developmental Editor: Shirley Kuhn
Designer: Maureen Sweeney
Production Manager: Peter Faber
Manuscript Editor: Janis Oppelt
Illustration Coordinator: Brett MacNaughton
Indexer: Kathleen Cole
Cover Designer: Brett MacNaughton

Doppler Ultrasound: Principles and Instruments   ISBN   0–7216–2864–8

Printed in the United States of America.

Last digit is the print number: 9   8   7   6   5   4   3   2   1

To Mom

Preface

Doppler Ultrasound: Principles and Instruments provides vascular technologists, sonographers, and physicians who need basic knowledge of the physical principles and instrumentation of doppler ultrasound with a simple explanation of how doppler ultrasound works. It does not describe how to perform diagnostic examinations or how to interpret the results, except in the consideration of spectral displays in Chapter 6 and artifacts in Chapter 7.

Exercises are provided in each chapter to check progress, strengthen concepts, and provide practice for registry and specialty-board examinations. Answers to all exercises are given beginning on page 234. A comprehensive multiple-choice examination with explanatory referenced answers is given in Appendix B.

The word doppler is not capitalized in this book because it is used as an adjective and not as a proper noun. This move, which may be considered bold by some, is not without precedent (e.g., the units hertz, ampere, joule, newton, watt, and ohm).

The author gratefully acknowledges stimulating and helpful discussions with his friend and former Yale colleague, Peter Burns, at Thomas Jefferson University and with David Phillips at the University of Washington, whose recent untimely death has saddened us all. He appreciates the continuing working relationship with his former Yale colleague, Ken Taylor, who has provided several images used in this book. He thanks Chris Merritt, Peter Burns, Rob Gill, Gene Strandness, David Taylor, Delores Pretorius, Abdel Nomeir, Terry Needham, and Cindy Burnham,

The American Institute of Ultrasound in Medicine, and the following companies: Acuson, Advanced Technology Laboratories, General Electric, Hewlett-Packard, Quantum Medical Systems, ATS Laboratories, JJ&A Instruments, Medisonics, Nuclear Associates, Nuclear Enterprises, and Radiation Measurements, Inc., for sharing several figures used throughout the book. The cover photograph was provided by Hewlett-Packard. He thanks Joe Roselli for artwork and Jo Patterson and Marie King for proofreading. He is particularly grateful to Louise Nixon for typing the entire manuscript.

FREDERICK W. KREMKAU, PHD

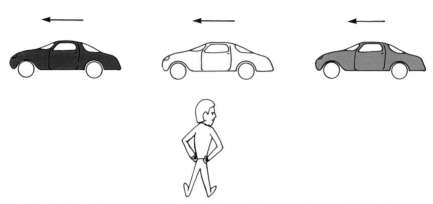

Color Plate I. A yellow automobile traveling at 15 percent the speed of light would appear blue as it approaches, yellow as it passes by, and red as it recedes.

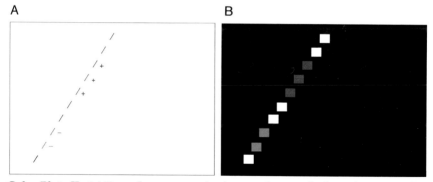

Color Plate II. (a) Ten echoes are received as a pulse travels through tissues. Three (red) have positive doppler shifts and two (blue) have negative shifts. (b) These are shown as red and blue pixels, respectively, on the color-flow display.

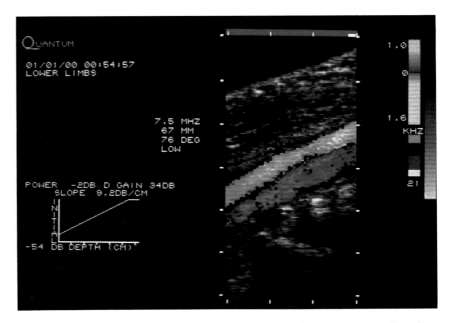

Color Plate III. Clinical example of color-flow doppler showing opposite flow directions in the two vessels. (Courtesy of Quantum Medical Systems.)

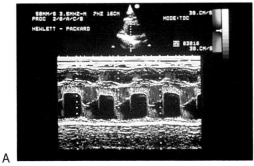

A

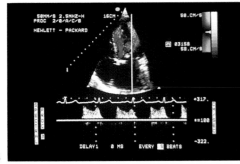

B

Color Plate IV. (a) Clinical example of color-flow doppler combined with M mode in the heart. (b) Clinical example of color-flow doppler combined with continuous-wave doppler spectrum in the heart. (Courtesy of Hewlett Packard.)

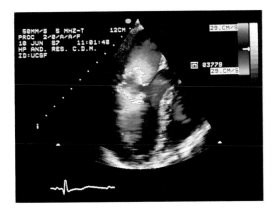

Color Plate V. Transesophageal cardiac color-flow image of the long axis in diastole. The blue colors between the left atrium and left ventricle represent blood traveling away from the transducer, but because of very high flow speeds, aliasing (Section 7.1) has occurred and the yellow and orange colors have replaced the blue colors. (Courtesy of Hewlett Packard.)

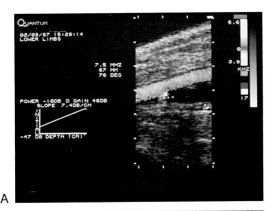

A

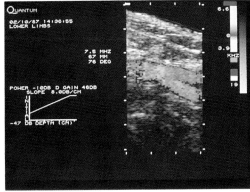

B

Color Plate VI. (a) Profunda branch off the femoral artery appears to have no flow (no color within it). (b) This view of the profunda shows color flow within it. The 90-degree doppler angle in (a) causes no doppler shift and lack of color. (Courtesy of CK Burnham.)

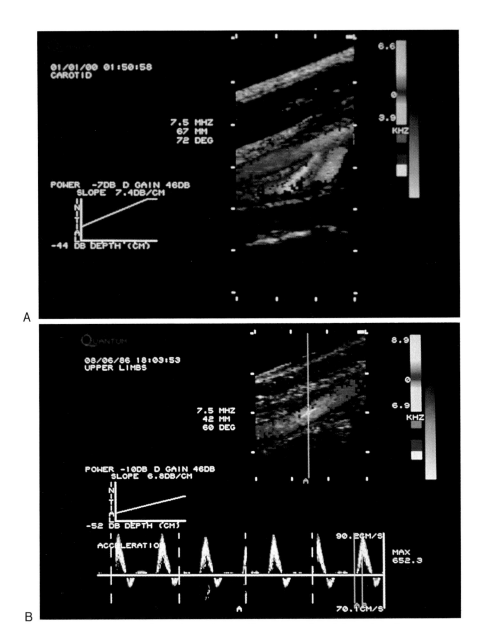

Color Plate VII. (a) Blue color indicates flow reversal and boundary layer separation in the carotid bulb. (b) Color flow in the brachial artery with spectral trace included. (Courtesy of Quantum Medical Systems.)

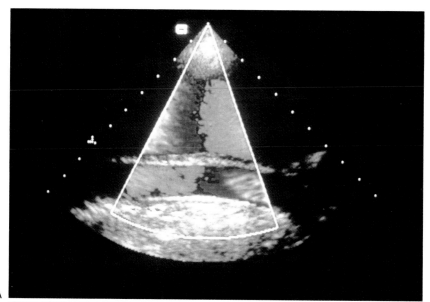

A

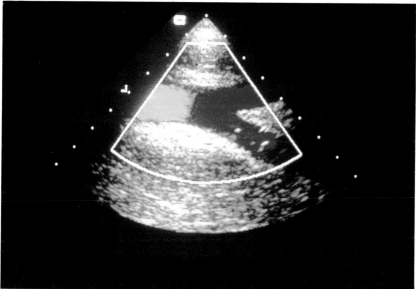

B

Color Plate VIII. (a) Color-flow presentation of aortic aneurysm (upper portion of image) and inferior vena cava (lower portion). (b) Color-flow presentation of the iliac bifurcation. (From Taylor KJW, Holland S: Doppler ultrasound I. Basic principles, instrumentation, and pitfalls. Radiology 174:297–307, 1990. Reprinted with permission. Courtesy of KJW Taylor.)

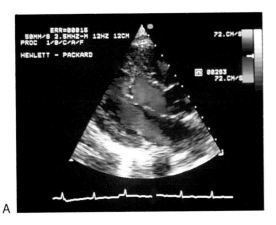

A

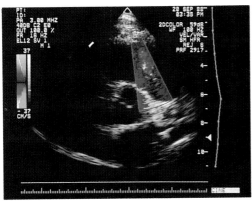

B

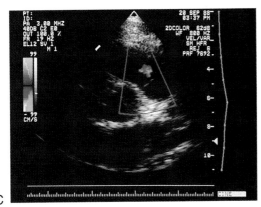

C

Color Plate IX. (a) Parasternal long-axis image of normal mitral-valve flow (courtesy of Hewlett Packard); (b) cardiac flow jet with wall filter set at 100 Hz; (c) wall filter set at 800 Hz (b and c courtesy of Advanced Technology Laboratories).

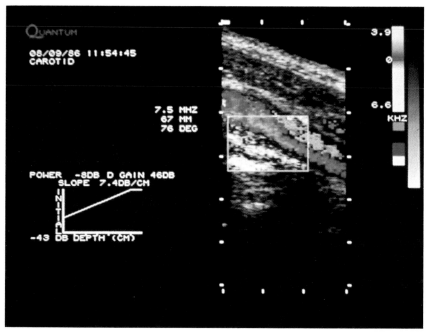

Color Plate X. Turbulent flow (blue) caused by carotid artery atheroma. (Courtesy of Quantum Medical Systems.)

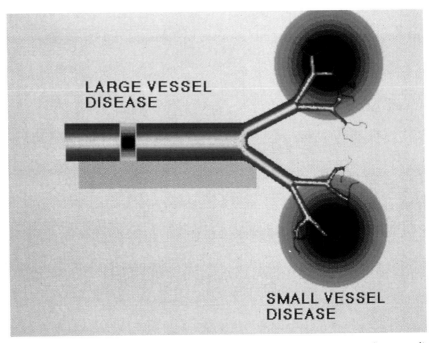

Color Plate XI. Doppler spectral displays provide information about flow conditions at the site of measurement and distal to it. (Courtesy of CRB Merritt.)

Contents

Chapter 1

Introduction

0717792625 22

The doppler effect was used by bats, dolphins, and other animals long before humans applied it to their needs. These animals make use of doppler information to determine motion of prey. Human applications of the effect have included those involving light, radar, and sound. Doppler shifts in light received from stars and galaxies have enabled us to conclude that the universe is expanding and to determine detailed motions of closer bodies such as the sun. The use of doppler radar in weather forecasting, aviation safety, and police highway surveillance has made the term a household word. As well as experiencing the acoustic doppler effect in normal everyday life (for example, approaching and receding sirens or vehicle horns), we have applied it in such uses as automatic door openers in public buildings and portable home burglar alarms.

Doppler ultrasound has been in use in medicine for many years. The primary long-standing applications include monitoring of the fetal heart rate during labor and delivery and evaluating blood flow in the carotid artery. Applications that have developed largely in the last decade have extended its use to virtually all medical specialties including cardiology, neurology, radiology, obstetrics, pediatrics, and surgery. Flow can be detected even in vessels that are too small to image. Doppler ultrasound

1

can determine the presence or absence of flow, flow direction, and flow character. For intelligent and successful application of the technique to medical diagnosis, an understanding of doppler physics is necessary.[1]

The early investigation into the nature of the effect about 150 years ago by Christian Andreas Doppler is an interesting story.[2-7] Because of his work, the effect is named after him. Note that his name is often given incorrectly as Johann in the scientific and medical literature. His father's name was Johann Evangialist Doppler.

The doppler effect is a change in frequency or wavelength due to motion. The motion can be that of the source, receiver, or a reflector of the wave. In medical applications it is commonly the motion or flow of blood that is the source of the doppler effect and about which information is desired. This diagnostic technique is accomplished as follows: Continuous-wave or pulsed-wave ultrasound is transmitted into the patient's body (Fig. 1.1a). Echoes are generated as the sound interacts with the tissues (Fig. 1.1b). Where echo-generating structures (heart and blood-vessel walls) or blood are moving, doppler-shifted echoes are generated. These echoes are received by a transducer and converted into electric voltages that pass into the electronics of the instrument. Here the voltages representing the echoes are amplified, and the doppler shift is determined. Doppler-shift frequencies representing motion or flow are applied to a loudspeaker for audible analysis and, commonly, to a display for visual analysis (Fig. 1.2). Pulsed-doppler instruments are often combined with pulse-echo imaging[8] to intelligently select and evaluate flow data (Fig. 1.2). More recently, rapid scanning and processing of doppler data have allowed two-dimensional, cross-sectional, real-time presentation of

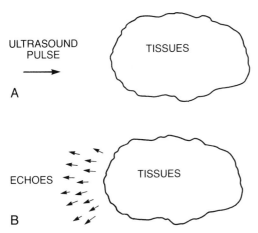

Figure 1.1. (a) In diagnostic ultrasound, ultrasound is sent into the tissues to interact with them and obtain information about them; (b) reflected and scattered ultrasound (echoes) return from the tissues, providing information useful for imaging, flow measurement, and diagnosis.

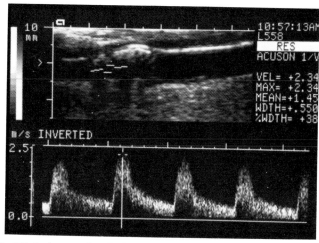

Figure 1.2. Clinical example of a linear scan with doppler blood flow information. (Courtesy of Acuson.)

doppler flow data superimposed on the real-time, gray-scale, cross-sectional anatomic image.

One of the fundamental limitations of flow information provided by the doppler effect is that it is angle dependent. Investigations are being carried out on nondoppler ultrasound approaches to flow measurement, which do not have this angle dependence.[9,10]

In this book we consider the following questions: How does ultrasound detect and measure flow? In what ways is flow information presented? How is flow detection localized to a specific site in tissue? How is two-dimensional flow determined and presented in real time? Other textbooks dealing with the physics of doppler ultrasound include References 11 through 13. Textbooks dealing with medical applications include References 13 through 22.

Exercises

1.1 The doppler effect is a change in (more than one correct answer)
  a. amplitude
  b. intensity
  c. impedance
  d. frequency
  e. wavelength

1.2 The change in Exercise 1.1 is a result of _____.

1.3 The motion producing the doppler effect can be that of the (more than one correct answer)

    a. source

    b. receiver

    c. memory

    d. display

    e. reflector

1.4 In medical applications, it is commonly the flow of _____ that is the source of the doppler effect. Doppler shift frequencies are applied to a _____ for audible analysis and commonly to a _____ for visual analysis.

1.5 A fundamental limitation of flow information provided by the doppler effect is its dependence on _____.

Answers to Exercises are given beginning on page 234.

Chapter 2

Sonography

The information in this chapter is important to the understanding of doppler ultrasound for two reasons. First, ultrasound (Section 2.1) and transducers (Section 2.2) are used in doppler ultrasound and must be understood. Second, sonography is combined with doppler ultrasound in many applications. Thus, an understanding of imaging instruments (Section 2.3) and artifacts (Section 2.4) is important.

Ultrasound imaging (sonography) is accomplished with a pulse-echo technique. Pulses of ultrasound (generated by a transducer) are sent into the patient (see Fig. 1.1a), where they produce echoes at organ boundaries and within tissues. These echoes return (see Fig. 1.1b) to the transducer, where they are detected and imaged. Thus, the transducer both generates the ultrasound pulses and detects the returning echoes. The ultrasound instrument processes this information and generates appropriate dots, which form the ultrasound image on the display. The brightness of each dot corresponds to the echo strength. The location of each dot corresponds to the anatomic location of the echo-generating structure. The positional information is determined by knowing the direction of the pulse when it enters the patient and measuring the time for its echo to return to the transducer. From an assumed starting point on the display (usually at the top) the proper location for presenting the echo can then be derived, knowing the direction in which to travel from that starting point to the appropriate distance. The ultrasound pulse and its echo are assumed to travel at 1.54 millimeters per microsecond (mm/μs) in tissues. This means that 13 μs are required for the ultrasound pulse to travel round trip to a structure located 1 centimeter (cm) away from the transducer (26 μs for 2 cm, 130 μs for 10 cm, and so forth).

If one pulse of ultrasound is transmitted into tissue or tissue-equivalent phantom material, a series of echoes will return as the pulse travels through the material. These get converted into a series of voltages (by the transducer) that are then processed by the electronics in the instrument and displayed as a string of dots on the display, i.e., one scan line (Fig. 2.1). If additional pulses are generated but each additional pulse has the same path, the same line is displayed over and over again (one repeating scan line). This is demonstrated in Figure 2.2, which shows an image (made with a stationary transducer) of a tissue-equivalent ultrasound phantom. If the process is repeated, but with different starting points for each subsequent pulse, a cross-sectional image begins to build up (Fig. 2.3). In this case, each pulse travels in the same direction but starts from a different point. This yields the parallel scan lines on the display in Figure

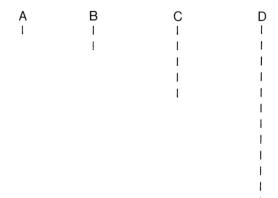

Figure 2.1. Echoes are presented in sequence on a scan line as they return from tissue as a pulse travels. (a) The first echo is displayed. (b) The second echo is added. (c) Three more echoes are added. (d) All the echoes from a single pulse have been received and displayed as a completed scan line. This would have occurred in less than 250 μs.

Figure 2.2. Image of a tissue-equivalent ultrasound phantom made with a stationary transducer (single-repeating scan line).

2.4. This partial cross-sectional image of a phantom (Section 7.2) has been produced with vertical parallel scan lines that are so close together that they cannot be identified individually. When the process is complete, a cross-sectional image of the phantom is produced (Fig. 2.5). The rectangular display resulting from this procedure is often called a linear scan. This is because the pulses originate from a line across the top of the scan, linear being the adjective form of line. A second approach to sending ultrasound pulses through the object to be imaged is shown in Figure 2.6. Here each pulse originates from the same starting point, but subsequent pulses go out in slightly different directions from previous ones. This results in a pie-shaped sector scan.

There are an unlimited number of scan formats. The linear and sector scans are the ones used most commonly in the automated scanning techniques described in Section 2.2. Others could be used, but, in each case, what is required is that ultrasound pulses be sent through all portions of the cross section that is to be imaged. Each pulse generates a series of echoes, which results in a series of dots or a scan line on the display. The resulting cross-sectional image is made up of many of these scan lines. The scan format determines the starting points and paths for the individual scan lines according to the starting point and path for each pulse used for

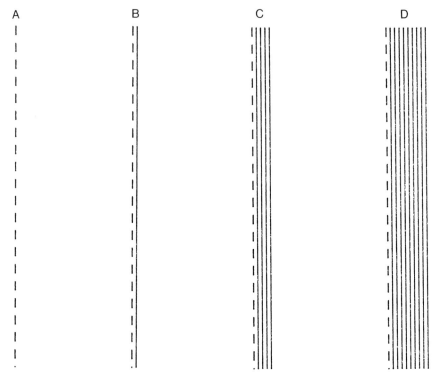

Figure 2.3. A single linear image or scan (frame) is made up of many scan lines; each represents a series of echoes returning from a pulse traveling through the tissues. (a) One scan line from one pulse as generated in Figure 2.1. (b) A second scan line is added. (c) Five and ten (d) scan lines.

generating each scan line. Figures 2.7 and 2.8 are examples of clinical cross-sectional ultrasound images of the linear and sector types, respectively. These are often called "B" scans. This terminology refers to the fact that the images are produced by scanning the ultrasound through the image cross section (i.e., sending pulses through all regions of the cross section) and converting echo strength into brightness of each represented echo on the display (thus "B" or brightness scan). Note that a B scan is an image of *echoes*, but it can be thought of as an image of anatomy since the imaged echoes are produced by the anatomy.

Continuous-wave or pulsed-wave ultrasound instruments may be combined with imaging instruments to yield what are commonly called duplex instruments. Figure 2.9 shows the flow in a vessel as a function of time (over several cardiac cycles). A cross-sectional image of the vessel is combined with indicators of the doppler beam location and region (sample

E

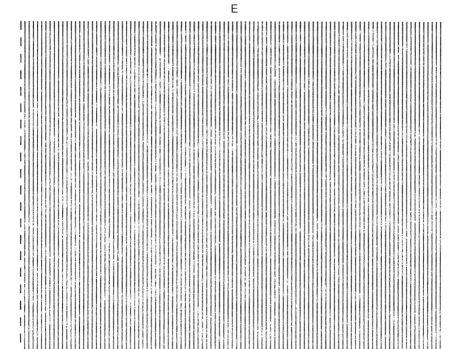

Figure 2.3 *Continued* (e) A complete linear frame consisting of (in this example) 100 scan lines. Less than 25 ms would be needed to display this frame. Thus, 40 such frames could be presented in sequence in a second of time.

volume) within the vessel from which the doppler information is being obtained. This will be discussed in greater detail in Chapter 5. Color-flow instruments also superimpose two-dimensional doppler information on anatomic B scans. Subsequent sections in this chapter deal with the primary aspects of sonography: ultrasound, transducers, instruments, and artifacts. Reference 8 gives more complete coverage of the material in this chapter.

2.1
Ultrasound

Ultrasound is like ordinary sound except that it has a pitch higher than what we can hear. Sound is a wave (i.e., a propagating or traveling variation in quantities called acoustic variables). These acoustic variables

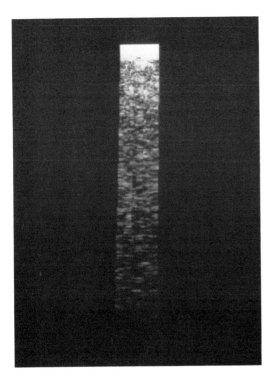

Figure 2.4 Partial linear scan of a phantom.

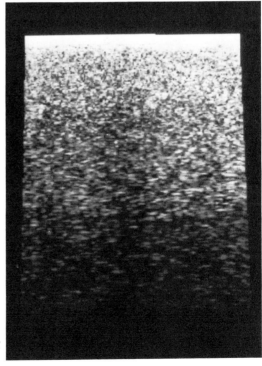

Figure 2.5. Complete linear scan of a phantom.

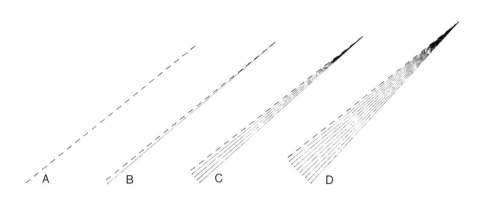

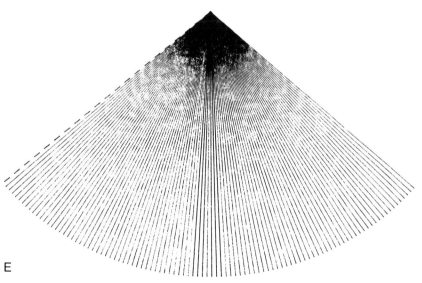

Figure 2.6. A single sector frame is built up by (a) one, (b) two, (c) five, (d) ten, and (e) 100 scan lines in sequence.

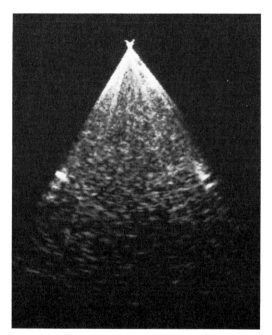

F

Figure 2.6 *Continued* (f) complete sector scan of a phantom.

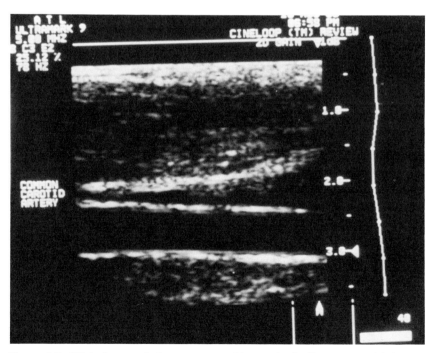

Figure 2.7. Clinical example (common carotid artery) of a linear scan with its rectangular shape. (Courtesy of Advanced Technology Laboratories.)

12

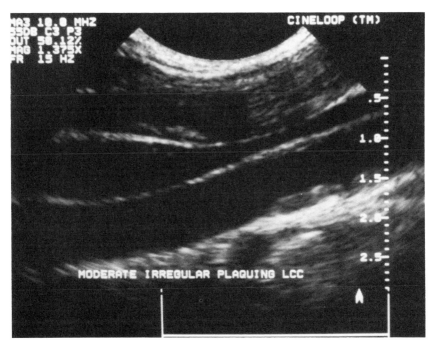

Figure 2.8. Clinical example (carotid artery plaque) of a sector scan with its pie-slice shape. (Courtesy of Advanced Technology Laboratories.)

include pressure, density, temperature, and particle motion. They go through repeating cycles of increase and decrease as the sound wave travels. Sound is a mechanical compressional wave in which back-and-forth particle motion is parallel to the direction of wave travel.

Frequency describes how many complete variations (cycles) an acoustic variable goes through in one second of time (i.e., how many cycles occur in a second). For example, pressure may start at its normal (undisturbed) value, increase to a maximum value, return to normal, decrease to a minimum value, and return to normal (Fig. 2.10). This describes a complete cycle of variation of pressure as an acoustic variable. As a sound wave travels past some point, this cycle is repeated over and over. The number of times that it occurs in 1 second is called the frequency. Frequency units include hertz (Hz) and megahertz (MHz). One hertz is one cycle per second and one megahertz is one million hertz. Sound with a frequency of 20,000 Hz or more is called ultrasound because it is beyond the frequency range of human hearing (the prefix ultra means "beyond").

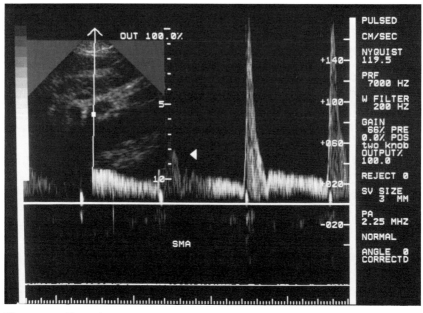

Figure 2.9. Clinical example (superior mesenteric artery) of a sector scan with doppler blood flow information. (Courtesy of Advanced Technology Laboratories.)

Wavelength is the length of space over which one cycle occurs (Fig. 2.11). If we could stop the sound wave, visualize it, and measure the distance from the beginning to the end of one cycle, the measured distance would be the wavelength.

Propagation speed is the speed with which a wave moves through a medium. It is the speed at which a particular value of an acoustic variable

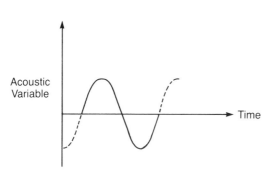

Figure 2.10. One complete variation (cycle) of an acoustic variable (e.g., pressure). This variation repeats as time passes, as indicated by the dashed lines. (From Kremkau FW: Basic principles and biological effects of ultrasound. *In* Resnick MI, Sanders RC: Ultrasound in Urology. Baltimore, Williams & Wilkins, 1979. Reprinted with permission.)

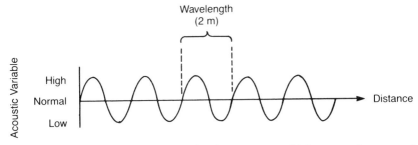

Figure 2.11. Wavelength is the length of space over which one cycle occurs. In this figure, each cycle covers 2 m. The wavelength is 2 m. For a propagation speed of 1.54 mm/μs and a frequency of 5 MHz, the wavelength is 0.3 mm.

moves or with which a cycle moves. Wavelength is equal to propagation speed divided by frequency.

$$\text{wavelength (mm)} = \frac{\text{propagation speed (mm/}\mu\text{s)}}{\text{frequency (MHz)}} \qquad \lambda = \frac{c}{f}$$

The average progagation speed in soft tissues (excluding lung and bone) is 1540 m/s or 1.54 mm/μs. Several others are listed in Table 2.1.

For sonography, short pulses of sound are used. This pulsed ultrasound is produced by applying electric pulses to the transducer. The number of pulses produced each second is called the pulse repetition frequency and is usually given in kilohertz (kHz). One kHz is 1000 Hz. The fraction of time the sound is on is called the duty factor.

Spatial pulse length is the length of space over which a pulse occurs (Fig. 2.12). It is equal to the wavelength times the number of cycles in the

Table 2.1
Propagation Speeds for Various Waves and Media (Miles per Hour)

Wave	Medium	Speed
Water surface	Water	20
Sound	Air	750
Sound	Water	3300
Sound	Tissue	3400
Light	Air	670,000,000

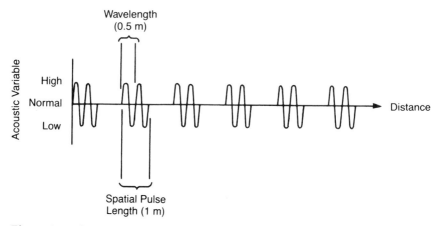

Figure 2.12. Spatial pulse length is the length of space over which a pulse occurs. It is equal to wavelength times the number of cycles in the pulse. In this figure, wavelength is 0.5 m; there are two cycles in each pulse, and spatial pulse length is 0.5 times 2 or 1 m.

pulse (typically two or three for imaging, more for doppler). Using the previous equation:

$$\text{spatial pulse length (mm)} = \frac{\text{number of cycles in pulse} \times \text{propagation speed (mm/}\mu s)}{\text{frequency (MHz)}}$$

$$\text{SPL} = \frac{nc}{f}$$

The strength of the ultrasound is described by two terms, amplitude and intensity. They would be measures of how loud the sound would be if it could be heard. Of course, it cannot be heard because it is ultrasound.

Amplitude is the maximum variation that occurs in an acoustic variable. It is the maximum value minus the normal (undisturbed) value (Fig. 2.13). Amplitude is given in units appropriate for the acoustic variable considered.

Intensity is the power in a wave divided by the area over which the power is spread.

$$\text{intensity (W/cm}^2) = \frac{\text{power (W)}}{\text{area (cm}^2)} \qquad I = \frac{P}{A}$$

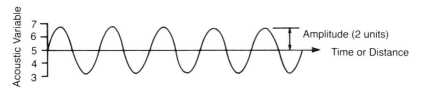

Figure 2.13. Amplitude is the maximum amount of variation that occurs in an acoustic variable. It is equal to the maximum value of the variable minus the normal (undisturbed) value. In this figure, the amplitude is seven (maximum value) minus five (normal value); the amplitude is two units.

Intensity is an important term in describing the sound that is produced and received by diagnostic instruments and in discussing bioeffects and safety. It may be illustrated by an analogy with sunlight incident on dry leaves (Fig. 2.14). Sunlight will not normally ignite the leaves, but if the same power is concentrated into a small area (increased intensity) by focusing with a magnifying glass, the leaves can be ignited. An effect is therefore produced by increasing the intensity even though the power remains the same. For our purposes, the area is the cross-sectional area of the sound beam discussed in Section 2.2.

Amplitude and intensity decrease as the sound travels through a medium. This reduction is called attenuation. It encompasses absorption (conversion of sound to heat), reflection, and scattering. Absorption is normally the dominant contribution to attenuation in soft tissue. Attenuation units are decibels (dB). The attenuation coefficient is the attenuation per unit length of sound travel. Its units are decibels per centimeter (dB/cm). The longer the path over which the sound travels, the greater the attenuation. The attenuation coefficient increases with increasing frequency. Persons who live in apartments or dormitories experience this fact when they hear mostly the bass notes through the wall from a neighbor's sound system. For soft tissues, attenuation coefficients are given by a simple proportional approximation of 0.5 dB of attenuation per cm for each MHz of frequency. Therefore, the average attenuation coefficient in dB/cm for soft tissues is approximately one-half the frequency in MHz. To calculate the attenuation in dB, simply multiply half the frequency in MHz (which is approximately equal to the attenuation coefficient in dB/cm) by the path length in cm, and the result is the attenuation in dB.

> attenuation (dB)
> $$= \frac{1}{2} \times \text{frequency (MHz)} \times \text{path length (cm)}$$
> $$a = \frac{1}{2}fL$$

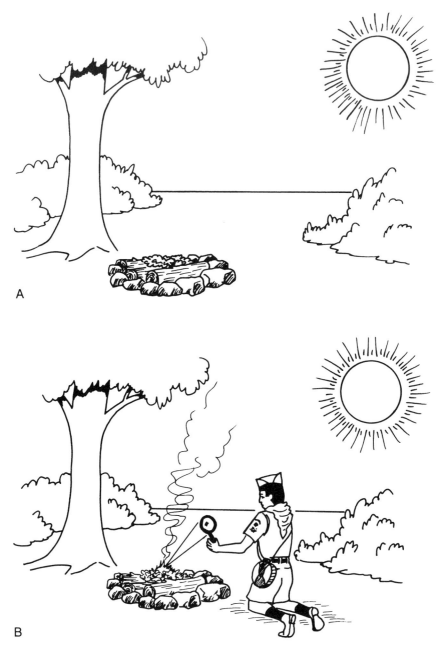

A

B

Figure 2.14. (a) Sunlight does not normally ignite a fire. (b) With focusing of the sunlight (increased intensity), ignition can occur.

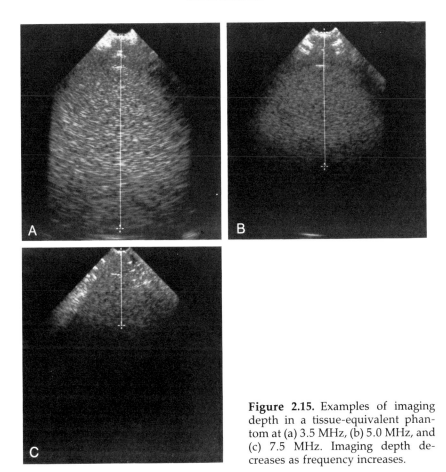

Figure 2.15. Examples of imaging depth in a tissue-equivalent phantom at (a) 3.5 MHz, (b) 5.0 MHz, and (c) 7.5 MHz. Imaging depth decreases as frequency increases.

A practical consequence of attenuation is that it limits the depth to which images and flow data can be obtained. As frequency is increased, attenuation increases, and imaging depth decreases (Fig. 2.15).

The usefulness of ultrasound as an imaging tool is primarily the result of reflection and scattering at organ boundaries and scattering within heterogeneous tissues. When an ultrasound pulse is incident on a boundary between two tissues, the incident sound may be reflected, transmitted, or both (Fig. 2.16a). The intensities of the reflected and transmitted sound depend on the incident intensity and the impedances of the tissue. Impedance is equal to density multiplied by propagation speed. If the two impedances are equal, there is no reflection and the transmitted intensity equals the incident intensity. The more different the impedances are, the stronger the reflected sound and the weaker the transmitted sound will be.

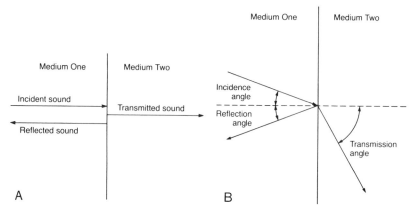

Figure 2.16. (a) Reflection and transmission at a boundary with perpendicular incidence. The lateral offset of transmitted and reflected sound with respect to incident sound is for figure clarity. An actual lateral shift does not occur. (b) Reflection and transmission at a boundary with oblique incidence. Incidence and reflection angles are equal. The transmission angle depends on the incidence angle and the media propagation speeds.

Oblique incidence occurs when the direction of travel of the incident ultrasound is not perpendicular to the boundary between two media (Fig. 2.16b). This is the common situation in diagnostic ultrasound. The direction of travel with respect to the boundary is given by the incidence angle. (For perpendicular incidence, the incidence angle is zero.) The reflected and transmitted directions are given by the reflection angle and transmission angle, respectively (Fig. 2.16b). They are related as follows:

reflection angle (degrees) = incidence angle (degrees) $\theta_r = \theta_i$

transmission angle (degrees) = incidence angle (degrees) ×

$$\left[\frac{\text{medium two propagation speed (mm/}\mu\text{s})}{\text{medium one propagation speed (mm/}\mu\text{s})}\right] \qquad \theta_t = \theta_i \left[\frac{c_2}{c_1}\right]$$

The second equation is the refraction equation. Refraction is a change in direction of sound when crossing a boundary (transmission angle unequal to incidence angle). The transmission angle is greater than the incidence angle if the propagation speed in medium two (c_2) is greater than the propagation speed in medium one (c_1). There is no refraction if the propagation speeds are equal.

Previously, we assumed that wavelength is small compared to the boundary dimensions and boundary roughness. The resulting reflections are called specular (mirror-like) reflections. If, on the other hand, the boundary dimensions are comparable to or small compared to the wavelength or if the boundary is not smooth (surface irregularities comparable in size to the wavelength), the incident sound will be scattered. Scattering is the redirection of sound in many directions by rough surfaces or by heterogeneous media (Fig. 2.17), such as tissues or particle suspensions like blood. These cases are analogous to light in which specular reflections occur at mirrors. For a rougher surface, such as a white wall, although virtually all the light is reflected (that is why the wall is white), a reflected image is not observed (as in a mirror) because the light is scattered at the surface and mixed up as it travels back to the viewer's eyes. When light passes through a suspension of water droplets in air (fog), it is scattered as well. Backscatter (sound scattered back in the direction from which it originally came) intensities vary with frequency and scatterer size. Normally, scatter intensities are much less than boundary specular reflection intensities. The intensity received by the transducer from specular reflections is highly angle dependent. Scattering from boundaries helps to make echo reception less dependent on incidence angle. Scattering, thus, permits ultrasound imaging of tissue boundaries that are not necessarily perpendicular to the direction of the incident sound. It also allows imaging of tissue parenchyma as well as organ boundaries. Scattering is relatively independent of the direction of the incident sound and therefore is more characteristic of the scatterers.

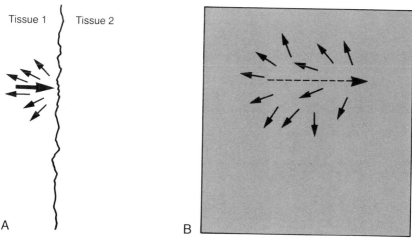

Figure 2.17. A sound pulse may be scattered by (a) a rough boundary between tissues or (b) from within tissues owing to their heterogeneous character.

The average speed of sound in tissues (1.54 mm/μs) leads to the important round-trip travel time rule of 13 μs/cm. That is, it takes 13 μs of round-trip travel time for each centimeter of distance from the transducer to the reflector or scatterer of sound. Thus, the deepest echoes (approximately 20 cm for abdominal imaging) will return approximately 250 μs after the pulse leaves the transducer.

2.2
Transducers

Transducers convert energy from one form to another. Ultrasound transducers have no special name, such as microphone or loudspeaker, which are the names applied to devices that accomplish similar functions with audible sound. Rather, they are simply referred to by the generic term, transducer. Ultrasound transducers convert electric energy into ultrasound energy and vice versa. Electric voltages applied to them are converted to ultrasound. Ultrasound (echoes) incident on them produce electric voltages. Ultrasound transducers operate on the piezoelectric principle, which states that some materials (ceramics, quartz, and others) produce a voltage when deformed by an applied pressure. Piezoelectricity also results in a production of a pressure when these materials are deformed by an applied voltage. Various formulations of lead zirconate titanate (PZT) are commonly used as materials for production of modern transducers. Ceramics such as these are not naturally piezoelectric (as quartz is). They are made piezoelectric during production by placing them in a strong electric field while they are at a high temperature.

Single-element transducers are in the form of discs (Fig. 2.18). When an electric voltage is applied to the faces, the thickness of the disc increases

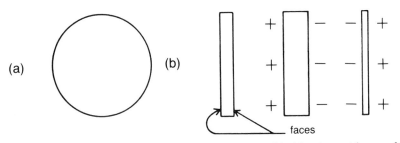

Figure 2.18. A disc transducer element. (a) Front view; (b) side view with no voltage applied to faces (normal thickness), voltage applied (increased thickness), and voltage of opposite polarity applied (decreased thickness).

Figure 2.19. A transducer assembly or probe. The damping material reduces pulse duration, thus improving axial resolution. The matching layer increases sound transmission into the tissues. The filler material enables the face of the transducer assembly to be flat. The transducer element is normally curved for focusing.

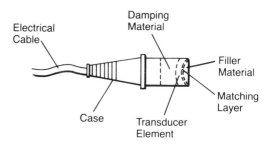

or decreases, depending on the polarity of the voltage. Transducer element (also called piezoelectric element, active element, or crystal) refers to the piece of piezoelectric material that converts electricity to ultrasound and vice versa. The element, with its associated case and damping and matching materials, is called a transducer assembly or probe (Fig. 2.19). Both the transducer element and the transducer assembly are commonly referred to as the transducer. Source transducers operated in the continuous mode are driven by a continuous alternating voltage and produce an alternating pressure that propagates as a sound wave (Fig. 2.20a). The frequency of the sound produced is equal to the frequency of the driving voltage. The operating frequency (sometimes called resonance frequency) of the transducer is its preferred frequency of operation. Operating frequency is determined by the thickness of the transducer element. The thinner the element is, the higher the frequency produced. This is analogous to the familiar fact that small bells produce a higher frequency sound than large ones. Continuous-wave sound entering a receiving transducer is converted to a

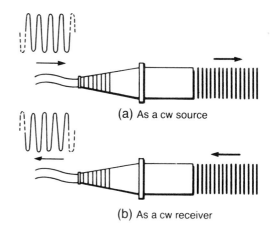

Figure 2.20. A transducer assembly operating in the continuous-wave mode. The device converts (a) a continuous wave voltage into continuous-wave ultrasound or converts (b) received continuous-wave ultrasound into a continuous-wave voltage.

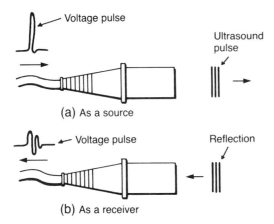

Figure 2.21. A transducer assembly operating in the pulsed mode. This device converts (a) electric voltage pulses into ultrasound pulses and converts (b) received ultrasound pulses (echoes) into electric voltage pulses.

continuous alternating voltage (Fig. 2.20b). For instruments employing the continuous-wave mode, separate source and receiver transducer elements are required, as they each must continuously perform their function. These elements are built into a single transducer assembly.

Source transducers operated in the pulsed mode (pulsed ultrasound) are driven by voltage pulses (see Section 2.3) and produce ultrasound pulses (Fig. 2.21). These transducers convert received reflections into voltage pulses. The pulse repetition frequency is equal to the voltage pulse repetition frequency, which is determined by the instrument driving the transducer. Damping material (a mixture of metal powder and a plastic or epoxy) is attached to the rear face of the transducer element to reduce the number of cycles in each pulse and thus the pulse length (Fig. 2.22). Reducing the pulse length improves resolution. This method of damping is analogous to packing foam rubber around a bell that is rung by a tap with a hammer. The rubber reduces the time that the bell rings following the tap. Typically, pulses of two or three cycles are generated with transducers used for sonography. Longer pulses are used with pulsed doppler instruments (Section 5.2).

A matching layer is commonly placed on the transducer face (Fig. 2.19). This material has an impedance intermediate between those of the transducer element and the tissue. It reduces the reflection of ultrasound at the transducer element surface, improving sound transmission across it in both directions (into and out of the tissues).

Because of its very low impedance, even a very thin layer of air between the transducer face and the skin surface will reflect virtually all the sound, preventing any penetration into the tissue. For this reason, a coupling medium, usually an aqueous gel or mineral oil, is applied to the

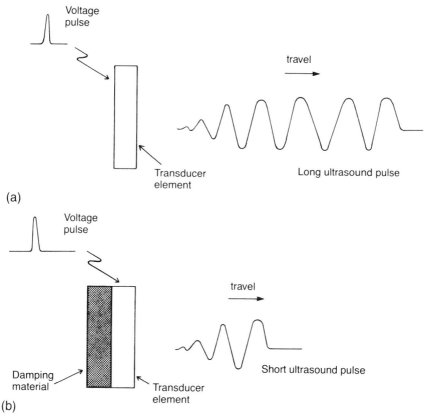

Figure 2.22. (a) Without damping, a voltage pulse applied to the transducer element results in a long pulse of many cycles. (b) With damping material on the rear face of the transducer element, application of a voltage pulse results in a short pulse of a few cycles. This figure shows each pulse traveling away from the transducer from left to right in space so that the right-hand end is the beginning or leading edge of the pulse.

skin before transducer contact. This eliminates the air layer and permits the sound to pass into the tissue.

A single-element flat disc transducer operating in the continuous-wave mode produces a sound beam with a beam diameter that varies according to the distance from the transducer face, as shown in Figure 2.23. Sometimes significant intensity travels out in some directions not included in the beam as pictured. These additional "beams" are called side lobes. They are really "cone" or "ring" beams for a disc transducer.

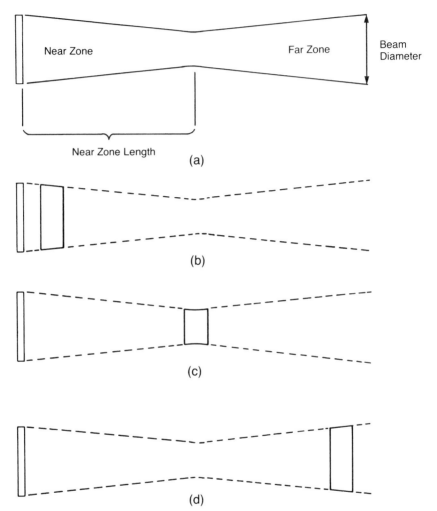

Figure 2.23. (a) Beam diameter for a single-element, unfocused disc transducer operating in the continuous-wave mode. This diameter approximates the region of that portion of the sound produced that is greater than 4 percent of the spatial peak intensity. The near zone is the region between the disc and the minimum beam diameter. The far zone is the region beyond the minimum beam diameter. Intensity is not constant within the beam, with intensity variations being greatest in the near zone. The beam diameter in (a) approximates the changing pulse diameter as an ultrasound pulse travels away from the transducer. (b) A pulse shortly after leaving the transducer. (c) Later the pulse is located at the end of the near-zone length, where its diameter is a minimum. (d) Still later the pulse is in the far zone, where its diameter is increasing as it travels. This figure assumes a nonscattering, nonrefracting medium such as water.

The region from the disc out to a distance of one near-zone length is called the near zone. The near zone is longer for larger diameter transducers and for higher frequency transducers. The region beyond a distance of one near-zone length is called the far zone. The beam diameter at any point depends on the frequency, transducer diameter, and distance from the transducer. It is important to realize that even for flat, unfocused transducer elements (Fig. 2.23), there is some beam narrowing or "focusing."

For improved resolution, beam diameter is reduced by focusing the sound in a manner similar to the focusing of light. Sound may be focused by employing a curved transducer element, a lens, or a phased array (Fig. 2.24). Focal length is the distance from the transducer to the center of the focal region. It cannot be greater than the near-zone length of the comparable unfocused transducer. Most diagnostic transducers are focused to some degree.

There are two ways in which automatic scanning of a sound beam can be performed: mechanical and electronic. Both of these methods provide a means for sweeping the sound beam through the tissues rapidly and repeatedly. The first method may be accomplished by oscillating a transducer in angle or by rotating a group of transducers (Fig. 2.25). In most mechanical real-time transducers, the rotating or oscillating component is immersed in a coupling liquid within the transducer assembly. The sound beam is thus swept at a rapid rate without movement of the entire transducer assembly.

Electronic scanning is performed with arrays. Transducer arrays are transducer assemblies with several transducer elements. The elements are

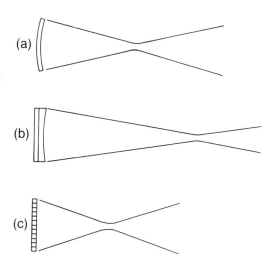

Figure 2.24. Sound focusing by (a) a curved transducer, (b) a lens, and (c) a phased array. Lenses focus because the propagation speed through them is higher than that through tissues. Refraction at the surface of the lens forms the beam such that a focal region occurs. The amount by which the beam diameter is reduced by focusing is described qualitatively as a weak or strong focus.

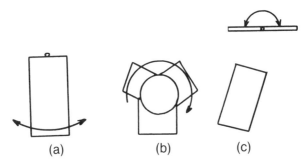

Figure 2.25. Mechanical real-time transducer types. (a) Oscillating transducer; (b) rotating group of transducers; (c) oscillating mirror (stationary transducer).

rectangular in shape and arranged in a line (linear array) or are ring shaped and arranged concentrically (annular array) (Fig. 2.26).

A linear-switched array (sometimes called a linear-sequenced array or simply a linear array) is operated by applying voltage pulses to groups of elements in succession (Fig. 2.27). The origin of the sound beam moves across the face of the transducer assembly and thus produces the same effect as manual linear scanning with a single-element transducer. Such electronic scanning, however, can be done in a more rapid and more consistent manner. If this electronic scanning is repeated rapidly enough, a real-time presentation of information can result. That is, several frames or images can be presented per second in rapid sequence.

A linear-phased array (commonly called a phased array) is operated

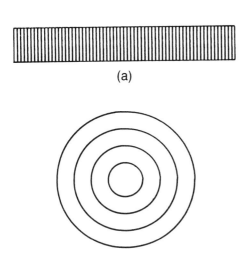

Figure 2.26. Front views of (a) a linear array with 64 rectangular elements and (b) an annular array with four elements.

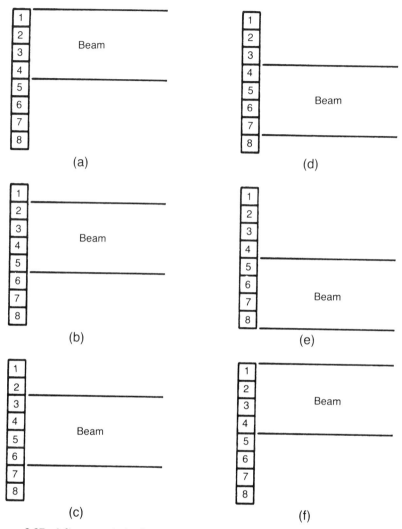

Figure 2.27. A linear-switched array (side view). Voltage pulses are applied simultaneously to all elements in a group: (a) first to elements 1 through 4 as a group, (b) next to elements 2 through 5, and (c–e) so on across the transducer assembly; (f) the process is then repeated.

by applying voltage pulses to all elements in the assembly as a complete group, but with small time differences (phasing), so that the resulting sound pulse may be shaped and steered (Fig. 2.28). If the same time differences are used each time the process is repeated, the same beam shape and direction will result repeatedly. However, the time differences may be

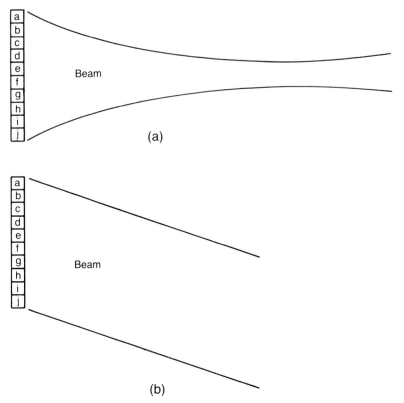

Figure 2.28. A linear-phased array (side view). (a) By applying voltage pulses to the upper and lower elements earlier than to the middle elements, the beam can be focused. (b) By applying voltage pulses to the upper elements earlier than to the lower elements, the beam can be steered down. Similarly, by applying voltage pulses to the lower elements earlier, the beam can be steered up. Pulses may be applied in such a way that parts (a) and (b) are combined, resulting in a focused and steered beam.

changed with each successive repetition so that the beam shape or direction (Fig. 2.29) can continually change. This can then result in sweeping of the beam (the beam direction changes with each pulse) and in variable focusing (the focal length changes with each pulse). Phased arrays can be of the linear array or annular array type. Annular arrays provide two-dimensional focusing, shaping the beam like an ice-cream cone. However, they must be mechanically scanned as shown in Figure 2.25a and c.

There are two primary aspects to resolution in imaging: detail (geometric) resolution and contrast (gray-scale) resolution. The latter is discussed in the next section and the former here. If two reflectors are not

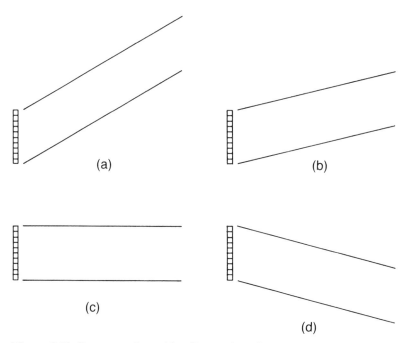

Figure 2.29. Beam steering with a linear-phased array. (a) The pulse is directed at an upward angle because the voltage pulse from the instrument pulser is applied to the elements in rapid succession from bottom to top. (b) The next pulse travels out at less of an upward angle because the time delays in applying the voltage pulse to the elements are less than in (a). (c) The next pulse travels out horizontally because the voltage pulse is applied simultaneously to all the elements. (d) The next pulse is directed at a downward angle because the voltage pulse is applied in rapid succession to the elements from top to bottom.

sufficiently separated, they will not produce separate reflections and thus will not be separated on the instrument display. Characteristics of the instrument's electronics and display may further degrade this detail resolution. It is apparent, however, that if separate reflections are not initially generated, the reflectors will not be separated on the display. In ultrasound imaging there are two aspects to detail resolution, axial and lateral. They depend on pulse length and pulse width, respectively. The shorter the pulse is, the better the axial resolution; the narrower the pulse is, the better the lateral resolution. Damping and use of higher frequencies shorten the pulse, improving axial resolution. Focusing narrows the pulse, improving lateral resolution (at least in the focal region). Axial resolution is equal to one half the pulse length. Lateral resolution is equal to pulse width. Both are like a golf score, the smaller the better. Improved resolu-

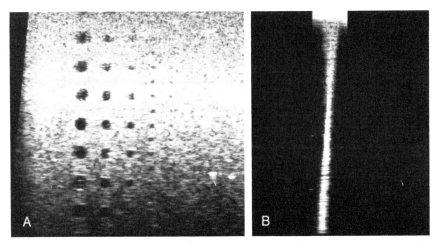

Figure 2.30. (a) An image of a resolution penetration phantom that contains circular anechoic regions ("cysts") in tissue-equivalent material (see Chapter 7). From left to right, the "cysts" are 10, 8, 6, 4, 3, and 2 mm in diameter and occur every 1 to 2 cm in depth. Close examination shows that the 3-mm "cysts" are the smallest that can be resolved, and they are visible only in the range of 5- to 11-cm depth. This image was produced using a 3.5-MHz transducer. The beam profile of this transducer is shown in (b). From this image, the focus appears to be at about 8-cm depth.

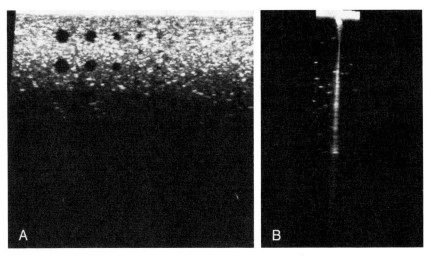

Figure 2.31 (a) The same phantom as in Figure 2.30(a) imaged with a 7.5-MHz transducer. In this instance, the 2-mm "cysts" can be seen in the first 4 cm of depth. This corresponds to the focal region of this transducer, as shown in (b) its beam profile. Also note in (a) that the imaging depth is substantially reduced compared with Figure 2.30(a). This reduction in imaging depth is due to the fact that the tissue attenuation increases with increasing frequency (3.5 MHz to 7.5 MHz). Detail resolution can be improved by increasing the frequency of the ultrasound beam but at the expense of decreasing the image depth.

tion with higher frequency (Figs. 2.30 and 2.31) is accompanied by decreased imaging depth due to increased attenuation (Section 2.1).

2.3
Instruments

Imaging systems produce visual displays from the electric voltages (representing echoes) received from a transducer. A diagram of the components of a pulse-echo imaging system is given in Figure 2.32.

The pulser is where the action originates. It produces electric voltage pulses (Fig. 2.33) that drive the transducer, which produces ultrasound pulses. The pulse repetition frequency of the pulser is the number of electric pulses produced per second. It is typically a few thousand hertz. Included in the functions of the pulser, when array transducers are used, is the production of delays and variations in pulse amplitudes necessary for the electronic control of beam scanning, steering, and shaping described in the previous section.

Voltages produced by the transducer in response to echoes are sent to the receiver for processing. The receiver performs amplification, compensation, and other functions[8] on these voltages representing the echoes.

Figure 2.32. The components of a pulse-echo imaging system. The pulser produces electric pulses that drive the transducer (T). It also produces pulses that tell the receiver and memory when the transducer has been driven. The transducer (acting as a source) produces an ultrasound pulse for each electric pulse applied. For each echo received from the tissues, an electric voltage is produced by the transducer (acting as a receiving transducer). These voltages go to

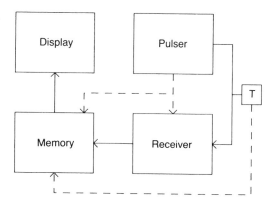

the receiver, where they are processed to a form suitable for driving the memory. Information on transducer orientation (which way it is pointing) is delivered (dashed lines) by electric voltages to the memory. Electric information from memory drives the display, which produces a visual image of the cross-sectional anatomy interrogated by the system. Some authors consider a clock or timing circuit separately in a diagram such as this. The clock determines the pulse repetition frequency and causes the various components of the instrument to work together. In this figure and in Section 2.3, the clock is considered to be part of the pulser.

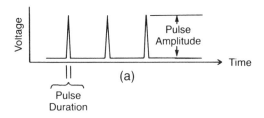

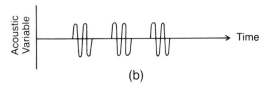

Figure 2.33. (a) For every voltage pulse applied, (b) an ultrasound pulse is produced by the transducer.

Amplification is increasing the small voltages received from the transducer to larger ones suitable for processing and storage. Receiver amplifiers usually have 60 to 100 decibels of gain.[8] Compensation (also called gain compensation, swept gain, time gain compensation [TGC], or depth gain compensation) equalizes differences in received reflection amplitudes because of reflector depth. Comparable reflectors will not result in equal amplitude reflections arriving at the transducer if their travel distances are different. (Distances from the transducer to the reflectors are different.) This is because attenuation depends on path length. It is desirable to display echoes from comparable reflectors in a similar way (comparable brightness). As these reflections may not arrive with the same amplitude, because of different path lengths, their amplitudes must be adjusted to compensate for path length differences. Larger path lengths result in later arrival times. Therefore, if voltages from reflections arriving later are amplified more than earlier ones, attenuation compensation is accomplished. This is what compensation does (Fig. 2.34). The rate of increase of gain as echoes return from a pulse is called the TGC slope.

Storing each cross-sectional image in memory as the sound beam is scanned through the tissue permits the display of a single image (scan) out of the rapid sequence of several images (frames) normally acquired each second in dynamic (real-time) ultrasound instruments. Displaying one scan out of the sequence is called freeze frame. Some instruments have enough memory to store the last several frames acquired; this is sometimes called "cineloop." Ultrasound instrument memories are commonly com-

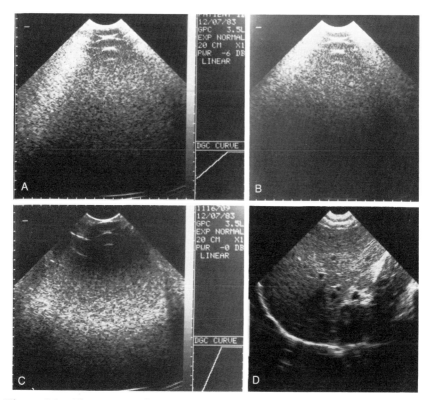

Figure 2.34. Three scans of a tissue-equivalent phantom imaged at 3.5 MHz with different settings of the time gain compensation (TGC). These scans show (a) correct compensation, (b) undercompensation, and (c) overcompensation; (d) a liver scan with proper TGC. Without TGC, the echo brightness (amplitude, intensity, strength) would fall off with depth (top to bottom).

puter memories that store the echoes in the form of numbers. They are called digital scan converters because they provide a computerized means for displaying a scan using a television scan format from information acquired by a linear or sector scanning technique. The image is divided into squares called pixels (picture elements), commonly 512 × 512 squares on each side. In each of these spaces a number is stored that corresponds to the echo intensity received from the point within the body corresponding to that storage position (Fig. 2.35). To image a gray scale (several shades of gray or brightness), it is necessary to have more than one checkerboard of memory. In a four-bit (binary digit) memory there are four checkerboards back to back so that each pixel has four bits associated with it (Fig. 2.36). Any pixel can store a number from 0 to 15 (16-shade system

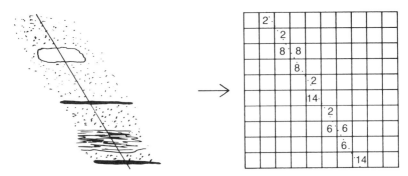

Figure 2.35. Anatomic cross-section scanned and front view of digital scan converter. Numbers are stored in the memory elements according to the intensity of the echoes received from corresponding anatomic locations.

in a four-bit memory). Other examples are given in Table 2.2. Eight-bit memories are now common in sonography.

The procedure for storing the information required for display of the two-dimensional, cross-sectional image for a digital scan converter is as follows: the beam is scanned through the patient in such a way that the ultrasound beam "cuts" through the tissue in a cross section. Echoes received from all points on this cross section are converted to numbers, which are stored at corresponding places in the digital memory. All the information necessary for displaying this cross-sectional image is then stored in memory. The information can then be taken out of memory and applied to a two-dimensional display in such a way that the numbers coming out of memory are displayed with corresponding brightnesses on the

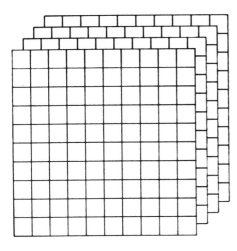

Figure 2.36. A 10 × 10 pixel, four-bit deep (four bits per pixel) digital memory.

Table 2.2
Characteristics of Digital Memories

Number of Bits	Lowest Number Stored	Highest Number Stored	Number of Shades
4	0	15	16
5	0	31	32
6	0	63	64
7	0	127	128
8	0	255	256

face of the tube (Fig. 2.37). An example of such a display is shown in Figure 2.38.

The display device is a cathode array tube. This tube generates a sharply focused beam of electrons that produces a bright spot on the phosphor-coated front face (screen) of the tube (Fig. 2.39). This spot can be moved across or up and down the face by applying voltages to deflection plates or electric currents to magnetic deflection coils. If the voltage or current is properly varied, the spot can be made to move across the face at constant speed. At the completion of this motion (i.e., when an image line is completed), the spot can be made to jump rapidly back and down slightly to begin the next line. B-mode operation causes a brightening of the spot for each echo. The greater the echo intensity (the larger the number in memory), the brighter the spot. Television monitors are commonly used as the display devices for ultrasound imaging instruments. A television monitor is a cathode ray tube in which a particular electron beam scanning format is utilized. The electron beam current is continually changed as the beam is scanned to provide varying brightness of the spot,

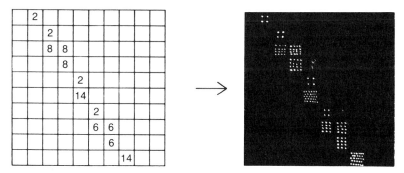

Figure 2.37. For display of scanned anatomic structures, numbers are read out of pixel locations in digital memory and applied to the display in such a way that brightness corresponds to the stored number.

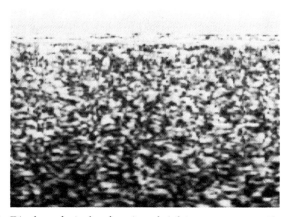

Figure 2.38. Display of pixels of various brightnesses representing various numbers in the corresponding memory locations. The display is magnified here to make the square pixels easily seen. Normally, they are too small and numerous to be noticed individually.

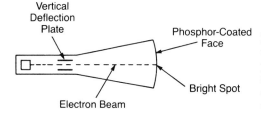

Figure 2.39. A cathode-ray tube (side view). The electron beam produces a bright spot where it strikes the phosphor-coated face of the tube. A set of horizontal deflection plates is not shown.

Figure 2.40. The television display format has 525 horizontal display scan lines, which are written out in one thirtieth of a second. Half of these (alternate solid lines) are written first, followed by the remaining

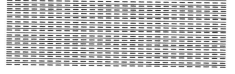

(dashed) ones. Each of these sets of lines (solid and dashed on this illustration) make up a "field." Two fields make a frame. Writing the frame in the format of two fields reduces flicker.

thus providing gray-scale imaging capability. The television scanning format consists of a left-to-right and top-to-bottom scanning pattern similar to the way in which this page of text is read. The resulting display consists of 525 horizontal display scan lines that produce one frame of a dynamic image (Fig. 2.40). This picture is updated (dynamic imaging) 30 times each second (real-time or dynamic imaging instruments must produce several cross-sectional images per second). This requires the use of mechanical or array real-time transducers (Section 2.2). Dynamic imaging provides rapid and convenient acquisition of the desired image (the display changes continuously as the beam is scanned through the tissues) and two-dimensional imaging of the motion of moving structures (the display continually changes as the structures move). Each complete scan of the sound beam produces an image on the display that is called a frame. Each frame is made of scan lines (one for each time the transducer is pulsed).

2.4
Artifacts

In imaging, an artifact is anything not properly indicative of structures imaged. It is caused by some characteristic of the imaging technique. Because some artifacts are useful, imaging can at times be better than direct viewing of the anatomy (if that were possible). This is because some ultrasound imaging artifacts, although errors from an anatomic imaging standpoint, give valuable information on the nature of objects or lesions that might not be apparent with other imaging methods or even direct viewing. In addition to helpful artifacts, there are several that hinder proper interpretation and diagnosis. These must be avoided or properly handled when encountered. Artifacts in ultrasound imaging occur as structures that are one of the following: not real, missing, improperly located, or of improper brightness, shape, or size.[8,23] Only five of eighteen known artifacts will be discussed here.

If two or more reflectors are encountered in the sound path, multiple reflections (reverberations) will occur. These may be sufficiently strong to be detected by the instrument and to cause confusion on the display. The process by which they are produced is shown in Figure 2.41. This results in placement on the image of reflectors that are not real. They will be placed beyond the second real reflector at separation intervals equal to the separation between the first and second real reflectors (Fig. 2.42).

Refraction can cause a reflector to be positioned improperly on the display (Figs. 2.43 and 2.44). A common site for this occurrence is in

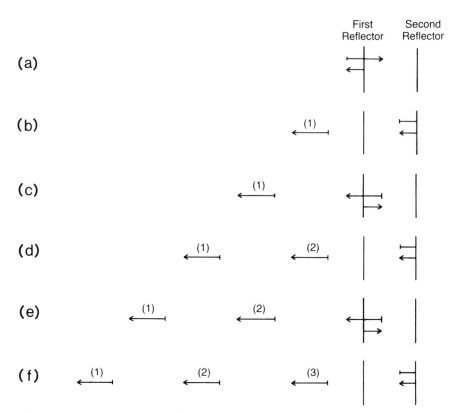

Figure 2.41. The generation of multiple reflections (reverberations). (a) An ultrasound pulse has come from the left, has encountered the first reflector, and has been partially reflected and partially transmitted. (b) Reflection and transmission at the first reflector are complete. Reflection at the second reflector is occurring. (c) Reflection at the second reflector is complete. Partial transmission (from right to left this time) and partial reflection are again occurring at the first reflector. (d) The reflections from the first (1) and second (2) reflectors are traveling to the left toward the sound source. A second reflection (repeat of [b]) is occurring at the second reflector. (e) Partial transmission and reflection are again occurring at the first reflector. (f) Three reflections are now traveling to the left: (1) is the reflection from the first reflector; (2) is the reflection from the second reflector; (3) is the reflection from the second reflector, reflected from the back side of the first reflector (c) and reflected again from the second reflector (d). A fourth reflection is being generated at the second reflector (f). Action proceeds from top to bottom in the figure. The first reflector is sometimes the transducer face.

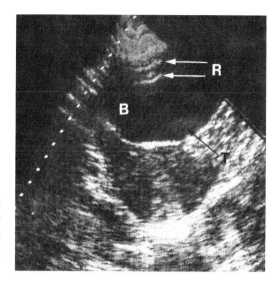

Figure 2.42. Reverberation (R) in the bladder (B). (From Kremkau FW, Taylor KJ: Artifacts in ultrasound imaging. J Ultrasound Med 5:227, 1986. Reprinted with permission.)

abdominal scanning with the transducer over the rectus abdominis muscle.

In a mirror image artifact, objects that are present on one side of a strong reflector are presented on the other side also (Fig. 2.45). This commonly occurs around the diaphragm (Fig. 2.46).

Shadowing is the reduction in echo amplitude from reflectors that lie behind a strongly reflecting (Fig. 2.47) or attenuating (Fig. 2.48) structure. Enhancement is the increase in reflection amplitude from reflectors that lie

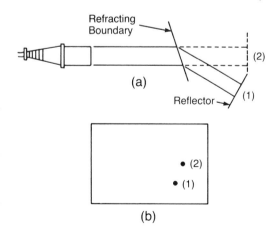

Figure 2.43. (a) Because of refraction, (b) improper positioning of the reflector occurs on the display. The system thinks the reflector is at position 2 because that is the direction in which the transducer is pointing. The reflector is actually at position 1.

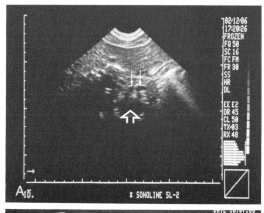

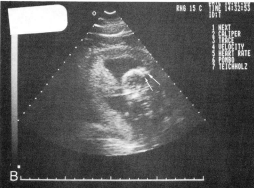

Figure 2.44. (a) Refraction (probably through the rectus abdominis muscle) has widened the aorta (open arrow) and produced a double image of the celiac trunk (arrows). (b) Refraction has produced a double image of a fetal skull (arrows).

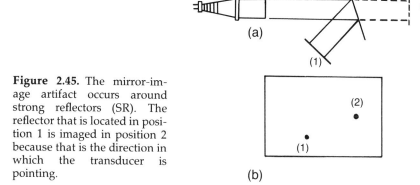

Figure 2.45. The mirror-image artifact occurs around strong reflectors (SR). The reflector that is located in position 1 is imaged in position 2 because that is the direction in which the transducer is pointing.

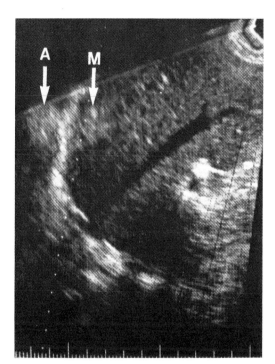

Figure 2.46. Anechoic mass (M) in the liver is also artifactually represented (A) superior to the diaphragm. (From Kremkau FW, Taylor KJ: Artifacts in ultrasound imaging. J Ultrasound Med 5:227, 1986. Reprinted with permission.)

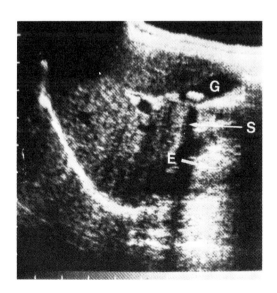

Figure 2.47. Shadowing (S) from a gallstone (G) and enhancement (E) from the gallbladder. (From Kremkau FW, Taylor KJ: Artifacts in ultrasound imaging. J Ultrasound Med 5:227, 1986. Reprinted with permission.)

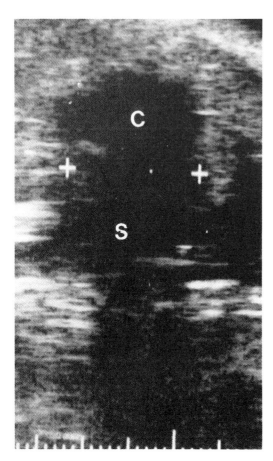

Figure 2.48. Anechoic breast carcinoma (C) with distal shadowing (S). (From Kremkau FW, Taylor KJ: Artifacts in ultrasound imaging. J Ultrasound Med 5:227, 1986. Reprinted with permission.)

behind a weakly attenuating structure (Figs. 2.47 and 2.49). Shadowing and enhancement result in reflectors being placed on the image with amplitudes that are too low and too high, respectively. Shadowing and enhancement are useful artifacts for determining the nature of masses.

2.5
Review

By sending short pulses of ultrasound into the body and using echoes received from tissue interfaces and from within tissues to produce images of internal structures, ultrasound is used as a medical diagnostic tool.

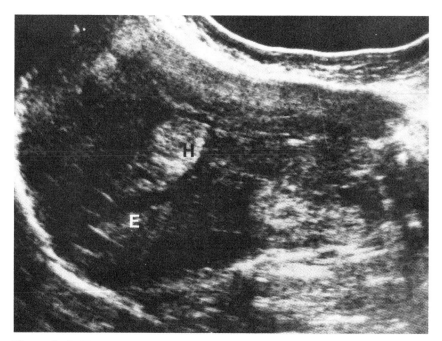

Figure 2.49. Hyperechoic hemangioma (H) with distal enhancement (E). (From Kremkau FW, Taylor KJ: Artifacts in ultrasound imaging. J Ultrasound Med 5:227, 1986. Reprinted with permission.)

Ultrasound is a wave of traveling acoustic variables described by frequency, wavelength, propagation speed, amplitude, intensity, and attenuation.

Pulsed ultrasound is used in sonography. It is described, additionally, by pulse repetition frequency and spatial pulse length. Diagnostic ultrasound commonly uses the frequency range of 2 to 10 MHz.

For perpendicular incidence at boundaries, reflections are produced if media impedances are different. For oblique incidence, refraction occurs if media propagation speeds are different. Scattering occurs at rough boundaries and within heterogeneous media. The distance to reflectors is found from the round-trip travel time.

Transducers convert electric energy to ultrasound energy and vice versa by piezoelectricity. Axial resolution is equal to one half the pulse length, which can be reduced (improving resolution) by damping and increasing frequency. Lateral resolution is equal to beam diameter, which can be reduced (improving resolution) by focusing. Disc transducers produce sound beams with near and far zones. Focusing can be accomplished only in the near zone of the comparable unfocused transducer. Arrays can scan, steer, and shape beams repeatedly, permitting dynamic imaging. Dynamic imaging can also be accomplished with mechanically driven single-element transducers or mirrors.

Pulse-echo systems use the amplitude, direction, and arrival time of echoes to produce images. Imaging systems consist of pulser, transducer, receiver, memory, and display. The pulser delivers the energizing voltages to the transducer, which responds by producing ultrasound pulses. Receivers amplify voltages representing returning echoes and compensate for attenuation. Digital memories store gray-scale image information and permit display on a television monitor. The number of bits per pixel in the digital memory determines the number of gray shades that can be displayed by the system. Dynamic imaging instruments display a rapid sequence of static pictures (frames).

Display artifacts include reverberation, refraction, mirror image, shadowing, and enhancement. The latter two are useful in evaluating masses producing them.

Exercises

2.1 The diagnostic ultrasound imaging method has two parts:
  1. Sending _____ of _____ into the body.
  2. Using _____ received from the tissues to produce an _____ of internal structures.

2.2 Ultrasound B scans are _____-_____ images of tissue cross sections.

2.3 The brightness of an echo, as presented on the display, represents its _____.

2.4 A linear scan is made up of many _____ scan lines.

2.5 A sector scan is made up of many scan lines with a common _____.

2.6 A linear scan has a _____ shape.

2.7 A sector scan is _____ shaped.

2.8 Sonography is accomplished by using a _____-_____ technique. The information of importance in doing this is the _____ from which the echo originated and the _____ of the echo. From these, the echo _____ and _____ on the display are determined.

2.9 Which of the following is a characteristic of a medium through which sound is propagating?

a. impedance
b. intensity
c. amplitude
d. frequency
e. period

2.10 Match the following:

_____ a. frequency	1. time per cycle
_____ b. period	2. maximum variation per cycle
_____ c. wavelength	3. length per cycle
_____ d. propagation speed	4. cycles per second
_____ e. amplitude	5. speed of a wave through a medium

2.11 If no refraction occurs as an oblique sound beam passes through the boundary between two materials, the _____ of the materials are known to be _____.

2.12 What must be known in order to calculate distance to a reflector?
a. attenuation, speed, density
b. attenuation, impedance
c. attenuation, absorption
d. travel time, speed
e. density, speed

2.13 With perpendicular incidence, if the impedances of two media are the same, there will be no
a. inflation
b. reflection
c. refraction
d. calibration
e. both b and c

2.14 No reflection will occur with perpendicular incidence if the media _____ are equal.

2.15 Scattering occurs at smooth boundaries and within homogeneous media. True or false?

2.16 Match the following transducer assembly parts with their functions:

_____ a. cable	1. reduces reflection at transducer surface
_____ b. damping material	2. converts voltage pulses to sound pulses
_____ c. piezoelectric element	3. reduces pulse duration
_____ d. matching layer	4. conducts voltage pulses

2.17 Which of the following improve sound transmission from the transducer element into the tissue? (More than one correct answer.)
a. matching layer
b. doppler effect

     c. damping material

     d. coupling medium

     e. refraction

2.18 Lateral resolution is improved by

     a. damping

     b. pulsing

     c. focusing

     d. reflecting

     e. absorbing

2.19 For a focused transducer, the best lateral resolution (minimum beam diameter) is found in the _____ region.

2.20 Beam diameter may be reduced in the near zone by focusing. True or false?

2.21 Beam diameter may be reduced in the far zone by focusing. True or false?

2.22 The axial resolution of a transducer can be improved most by

     a. increasing the damping

     b. increasing the diameter

     c. decreasing the damping

     d. decreasing the frequency

     e. decreasing the diameter

     f. attaching a dopple

2.23 The principle on which ultrasound transducers operate is the

     a. doppler effect

     b. acousto-optic effect

     c. acoustoelectric effect

     d. cause and effect

     e. piezoelectric effect

2.24 The lower and upper limits of the frequency range useful in diagnostic ultrasound are determined by _____ and _____ _____ requirements, respectively.

2.25 The range of frequencies useful for diagnostic ultrasound is _____ to _____ MHz.

2.26 The compensation (i.e., swept gain, and so forth) control

     a. compensates for machine instability in the warm-up time

     b. compensates for attenuation

     c. compensates for transducer aging and the ambient light in the examining area

     d. decreases the patient examination time

2.27 A gray-scale display shows

     a. gray color on a white background

     b. reflections with one brightness level

    c. a white color on a gray background

    d. a range of reflection amplitudes

2.28 A digital scan converter is a _____.

    a. compressor

    b. receiver

    c. display

    d. computer memory

    e. none of the above

2.29 Television displays produce _____ frames per second with _____ lines in each.

    a. 30, 60

    b. 30, 525

    c. 60, 512

    d. 512, 512

    e. 60, 120

2.30 In a digital instrument, echo intensity is represented by

    a. positive charge distribution

    b. a number stored in memory

    c. electron density of the scan converter writing beam

    d. a and c

    e. all of the above

2.31 If there were no attenuation in tissue, _____ would not be needed.

    a. rejection

    b. compression

    c. demodulation

    d. compensation

2.32 Reflection imaging includes ultrasound generation, propagation and reflection in tissues, and reception of returning _____.

2.33 Sonography instruments look for three things: the _____, _____, and arrival _____ of reflections that occur in tissues.

2.34 Imaging systems produce a visual _____ from the electric _____ received from the transducer.

2.35 The transducer is connected to the memory through the _____.

2.36 The transducer receives voltages from the _____ in pulse-echo systems.

2.37 The _____ receives voltages from the transducer.

2.38 Increasing gain generally produces the same effect as

    a. decreasing attenuation

    b. increasing attenuation

    c. increasing compression

    d. increasing rectification

    e. both b and c

2.39 Voltage pulses occur at the output of the

    a. pulser

    b. transducer

    c. receiver

    d. display

    e. both a and b

    f. both c and e

2.40 Ultrasound pulses from the pulser are applied to the

    a. pulser

    b. transducer

    c. receiver

    d. display

2.41 Gain and attenuation are usually given in

    a. dB

    b. dB/cm

    c. cm

    d. cm/3 dB

    e. none of the above

2.42 Compensation (swept gain) makes up for the fact that reflections from deeper reflectors arrive at the tranducer with greater amplitude. True or false?

2.43 A real-time B-mode display may be produced by rapid _____ transducer scanning or by _____ scanning of a transducer array.

2.44 Each complete scan of the sound beam produces an image on the display that is called a _____.

2.45 The number of lines in each frame is equal to the number of times the transducer is _____ while the frame is produced (while the sound beam is scanned).

2.46 Real-time imaging permits imaging of the motion of moving structures, but it is not as convenient as static B-mode imaging for acquiring desired static (freeze-frame) images. True or false?

2.47 In order to correct for attenuation, the TGC must (increase or decrease) _____ the amplification (gain) for increasing depth.

2.48 If a higher frequency is used, resolution is (improved or worsened), imaging depth (increases or decreases), and TGC slope must be (increased or decreased)?

2.49 Although dynamic imaging does not require a memory, most real-time scanners have one. It is necessary in order to have _____ _____ capability.

2.50 If a real-time scanner produces 1000 pulses per second and 20 frames per second, how many scan lines make up each frame?

2.51 Which of the following can cause improper location of objects on a display? (More than one correct answer.)
  a. shadowing
  b. enhancement
  c. reverberation
  d. mirror image
  e. refraction

2.52 Match these artifact causes with their results:
  _____ **a.** reverberation   **1.** unreal structure displayed
  _____ **b.** shadowing   **2.** structure displayed with
  _____ **c.** enhancement   improper brightness

2.53 Reverberation results in added reflectors being imaged with equal
  _____.

2.54 In reverberation, subsequent reflections are _____ than previous ones.

2.55 Enhancement is caused by a
  a. strongly reflecting structure
  b. weakly attenuating structure
  c. strongly attenuating structure
  d. refracting boundary
  e. propagation speed error

2.56 Shadowing results in decreased reflection amplitudes. True or false?

2.57 Which artifact should be suspected if observing twin gestational sacs when scanning through the rectus abdominis muscle?

Chapter 3

Hemodynamics

The word hemodynamics is derived from two Greek words meaning blood and power. The word thus refers to the forces and motion of blood flow and the science concerned with the study of blood circulation. An associated word is rheology, the science dealing with deformation and flow of matter. It comes from the Greek word rhein, meaning to flow.

Doppler ultrasound is used primarily for detecting and evaluating blood flow in the body. It is, therefore, important to understand the principles of this flow in order to effectively use this diagnostic tool.

The circulatory system consists of the heart, arteries, arterioles, capillaries, venules, and veins containing about 5 liters of blood. Flow in the heart, arteries, and veins can be detected with doppler ultrasound. The capillaries are the tiniest (a few micrometers in diameter) vessels. There are approximately 1 billion of them in the human body. It is across their walls that the exchange of gases and nutrients takes place with the body's cells. In this chapter we will consider the characteristics of fluids, such as blood, and their behavior when they flow through tubes, such as blood vessels, in steady and pulsatile flow forms.[24–28]

3.1
Fluids

Matter is generally classified into three categories: gas, liquid, and solid. Gases and liquids are fluids—substances that flow and conform to the shape of their containers. To flow is to move in a stream, continually changing position and possibly direction. Rivers flow downstream. Water flows through a garden hose. Air flows through a fan. Blood flows through the heart, arteries, capillaries, and veins.

Blood is a liquid (therefore a fluid) whose function is to supply nutrients and oxygen to the cells of the body and remove their waste products. Blood is a body tissue—a group of similar cells specialized to perform certain functions. It is made up of plasma, erythrocytes, leukocytes, and platelets. Plasma is primarily water (approximately 90 percent) and proteins. About 40 percent of blood volume is cells. This percentage is called hematocrit. Erythrocytes are the dominant (about 99 percent) cells in circulation. They contain hemoglobin, which is responsible for the transport of oxygen. Leukocytes are larger than erythrocytes but less numerous in blood. Their chief function is to protect the body against disease organisms. Platelets are smaller than erythrocytes and are important in the process of blood clotting.

Two important characteristics of fluids are density and viscosity. The density of a fluid is its mass per unit volume, commonly given in grams per milliliter (g/mL). Mass is a measure of an object's resistance to acceleration. This resistance is called inertia. The greater the mass, the greater the inertia. If two different masses are to be accelerated at the same rate, more force must be applied to the greater mass. The density of blood (1.05 g/mL) is slightly greater than that for water (1 g/mL) owing to the presence of proteins and cells. Viscosity is the resistance to flow offered by the fluid in motion. It is given in units of poise (honoring Poiseuille) or kg/m·s. One poise is one g/cm·s or 0.1 kg/m·s. Water has a relatively low viscosity (0.010 poise at 20°C and 0.0069 at 37°C) while that of molasses is high. The viscosity of blood plasma is about 50 percent greater than that

Table 3.1
Blood Properties

Density	1.05 g/mL
Viscosity	0.035 poise
Kinematic viscosity	0.033 stoke
Sound speed	1.57 mm/μs
Impedance	1.62 Mrayl
Attenuation	0.21 dB/cm·MHz

of water. The viscosity of normal blood is 0.035 poise at 37°C, approximately five times that of water. Blood viscosity can vary from about 0.02 (with anemia) to about 0.10 (with polycythemia). It also varies with flow speed. The viscosity divided by the density is a sometimes useful quantity that is given the name kinematic viscosity. For blood, its value is about 0.033 stoke. One stoke is one cm^2/s or 0.0001 m^2/s. Several properties of blood are listed in Table 3.1.

3.2
Steady Flow

Pressure is the driving force behind fluid flow. Pressure is force per unit area. It is equally distributed throughout a static fluid and exerts its force in all directions (Fig. 3.1). A pressure *difference* is required for flow to occur. Equal and opposite pressures applied at both ends of a liquid-filled tube will result in no flow. If the pressure is greater at one end than it is at the other, the liquid will flow from the higher pressure end to the lower pressure end. This pressure difference can be generated by a pump—for example, the heart in the circulatory system—or by the force of gravity, that is, by raising one end of a tube above the other. The greater the pressure difference, the greater the flow will be. This pressure difference is sometimes called a pressure gradient, although, strictly, pressure gradient is the pressure difference divided by the distance between the two pressure locations. Gradient comes from grade and refers to the

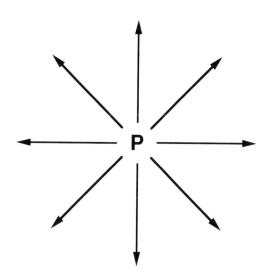

Figure 3.1. Pressure (P) is uniformly distributed throughout a static fluid and exerts its force in all directions.

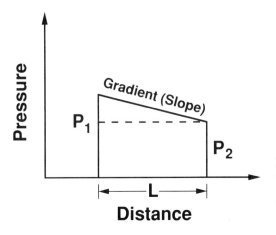

Figure 3.2. Pressure gradient or slope is the pressure difference ($P_1 - P_2$) divided by the separation (L) between the two pressure locations.

upward or downward sloping of something. As the pressure drops from one end of the tube to the other, this decrease can be thought of as a slope (i.e., the pressure difference divided by the distance over which the pressure drop occurs) (Fig. 3.2). In this section we consider a constant driving pressure that produces steady flow (unchanging with time). The driving pressure produced by the heart varies with time. This will be considered in Section 3.4.

The flow in a tube is determined not only by the pressure difference but also by the resistance to flow.

$$\text{volume flow (mL/s)} = \frac{\text{pressure difference (dyne/cm}^2)}{\text{flow resistance (g/cm}^4\cdot\text{s})} \qquad Q = \frac{\Delta P}{R}$$

This relationship between pressure and flow is known as Poiseuille's law. Flow here is volume flow (i.e., the volume of blood passing a point in a unit of time, usually given in milliliters (mL) per minute or per second). The total adult blood flow (cardiac output) is about 5000 mL/minute (i.e., the total blood volume circulates in about 1 minute). The flow resistance depends upon the fluid viscosity and the tube length and radius as follows:

$$\text{flow resistance} = \frac{8 \times \text{length} \times \text{viscosity}}{\pi \times \text{radius}^4} \qquad R = \frac{8L\nu}{\pi r^4}$$

As expected, an increase in viscosity or tube length increases the resistance and an increase in the size (radius or diameter) of the tube decreases the resistance. The latter effect is particularly strong, the resistance depending on the radius.[4] Thus, doubling the radius of a tube decreases its resistance to one sixteenth of the original value. By experience, we know that a longer or smaller diameter garden hose reduces water flow.

Substituting the equation for flow resistance into Poiseuille's law yields:

$$\text{volume flow} = \frac{\text{pressure difference} \times \pi \times \text{radius}^4}{8 \times \text{length} \times \text{viscosity}} \qquad Q = \frac{\Delta P \pi r^4}{8 L \nu}$$

Using tube diameter rather than radius yields:

$$\text{volume flow} = \frac{\text{pressure difference} \times \pi \times \text{diameter}^4}{128 \times \text{length} \times \text{viscosity}} \qquad Q = \frac{\Delta P \pi d^4}{128 L}$$

Units for these equations are dynes/cm² for pressure; cm for radius, diameter, and length; poise for viscosity; and milliliters per second for volume flow.

At the entrance to a tube the speed of the fluid is essentially constant across the tube (Fig. 3.3). This is called plug flow. After some distance, which depends upon the tube diameter, the average flow speed, and the viscosity, laminar flow is achieved (see Fig. 3.3). Laminar flow is a flow condition in which stream lines (describing fluid particle motion) are parallel to each other and to the tube walls. There is maximum flow speed at

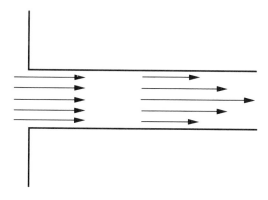

Figure 3.3. At the entrance to a tube or vessel, plug flow exists. After some distance, laminar flow is achieved.

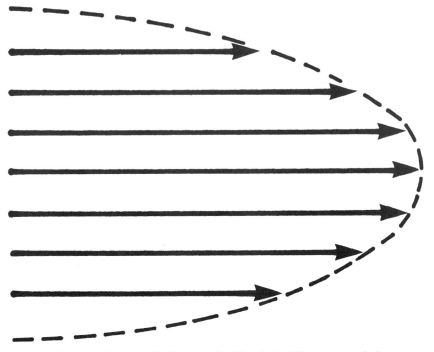

Figure 3.4. Parabolic flow profile. The dashed line is a parabola.

the center of the tube and minimum or zero flow at the tube walls. A decreasing profile of flow speeds from center to wall exists. Successive cylindrical layers (laminae) of fluid slide on each other with relative motion. The pressure difference at the ends of the tube overcomes the viscous resistance to this relative motion, maintaining the laminar flow through the tube. A parabolic flow profile results (Fig. 3.4). This means that the pattern of varying flow speeds across the tube is in the shape of a parabola (dashed line in Fig. 3.4). For parabolic flow, the average flow speed across the vessel is equal to one half the maximum flow speed (at the center).

> average flow speed
> $$= \tfrac{1}{2} \times \text{maximum flow speed} \qquad v_a = \tfrac{1}{2} \times v_m$$

Plug flow is found in larger vessels (e.g., the aorta), especially in systole. Parabolic flow is found in smaller vessels (e.g., the ovarian artery), especially in diastole. Combined flow character is found in intermediate-size vessels, such as the common carotid artery.

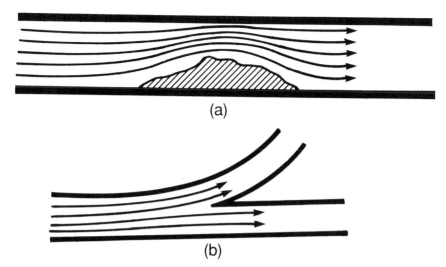

Figure 3.5. Disturbed flow at (a) a stenosis and at (b) a bifurcation.

Steady flow can be divided into three categories: laminar, disturbed, and turbulent. Laminar flow was discussed in the previous paragraph. Disturbed flow occurs when the parallel stream lines describing the flow are disturbed (Fig. 3.5). This occurs, for example, in the region of stenoses (next section) or at a bifurcation (splitting of a vessel into two). In disturbed flow, particles of fluid still flow generally in the forward direction. In the final category, turbulent flow, the flow pattern becomes random and chaotic with particles flowing in all directions, yet maintaining a net forward flow (Fig. 3.6). As flow speed increases in a tube, turbulent flow will eventually result (Fig. 3.6a). The onset of turbulent flow is predicted by the reynolds number, which has no units.

reynolds number

$$= \frac{\text{average flow speed} \times \text{tube diameter} \times \text{density}}{\text{viscosity}}$$

$$\mathrm{Re} = \frac{v_a \times d \times \rho}{\nu}$$

If the reynolds number exceeds about 2000 to 2500 (depending on tube geometry), flow becomes turbulent. With the exception of the heart and proximal aorta, turbulent flow does not normally occur in human circulation. Turbulent flow can also occur beyond an obstruction (Fig. 3.6b), such as a stenosis.

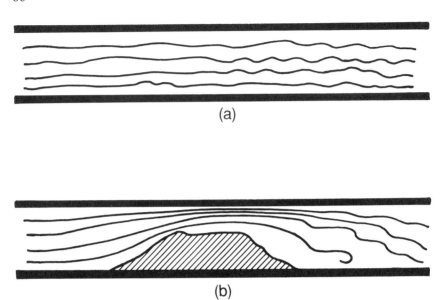

(a)

(b)

Figure 3.6. Turbulent flow in a vessel resulting from (a) too great a flow speed or (b) an obstruction.

3.3
Stenoses

A narrowing of a tube or vessel (stenosis) produces disturbed (see Fig. 3.5a), and possibly turbulent, flow (see Fig. 3.6b). The average flow speed in the stenosis must be greater than proximal and distal to it so that the volume flow can be constant throughout the tube. Examples of increased flow speed at a stenosis and turbulence beyond it are given in Figure 6.6. Volume flow must be constant for the three regions—proximal, at stenosis, and distal (continuity rule). This is because fluid is neither created nor destroyed as it flows through the tube. Volume flow is equal to average flow speed multiplied by the cross-sectional area of the flow (tube).

$$\text{volume flow} = \text{average speed} \times \text{tube area} \qquad Q = v_a \times A$$

Therefore, if the stenosis has an area one half that of the proximal and distal tube, the average flow speed within the stenosis must be double that proximal and distal to it. The above equation is known as the continuity equation. An analogy to this is traffic flow on a multilane highway (Fig.

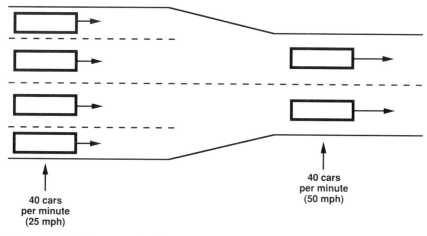

Figure 3.7. Highway traffic flow analogy to fluid volume flow. In the four-lane portion of the highway, 40 cars pass by each minute at a speed of 25 miles per hour. In the two-lane region, in order to maintain the (volume) flow of 40 cars per minute, a speed of 50 miles per hour is required. In this case, the speed times the number of lanes must be constant (100 lane-miles per hour). This is analogous to fluid volume flow in which tube cross-sectional area times flow speed must be constant.

3.7). In order to maintain volume flow (vehicles past a point per unit time), the vehicles must travel faster in the narrow region.

The cross-sectional area of a circular tube is:

$$\text{area} = \pi \times \text{radius}^2 \qquad A = \pi \times r^2$$

If the stenosis has diameter one half that adjacent to it, the area at the stenosis is one fourth that adjacent to it, and the average flow speed in the stenosis must quadruple.

Poiseuille's equation converted to average flow speed rather than volume flow is:

$$\text{average speed} = \frac{\text{pressure difference} \times \text{radius}^2}{8 \times \text{length} \times \text{viscosity}} \qquad v_a = \frac{\Delta P r^2}{8 L \nu}$$

This form of the pressure-flow relationship is particularly useful because doppler shift (Section 4.1) is proportional to flow speed, not volume flow (volume flow must be calculated from flow speed measurements (Section

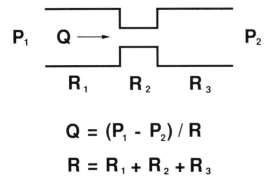

P_1 Q $\longrightarrow$ P_2

R_1 R_2 R_3

$Q = (P_1 - P_2) / R$

$R = R_1 + R_2 + R_3$

Figure 3.8. The overall flow resistance (R) for a vessel with a stenosis is equal to the sum of the resistances of the three parts (proximal [R_1], stenosis [R_2], and distal [R_3]). Volume flow (Q) is equal to the pressure difference at the ends of the vessel divided by the total resistance.

5.2). We see that flow speed (and, therefore, doppler shift) increases with tube radius (or diameter) squared. In summary, volume flow depends on radius to the fourth power, while flow speed depends on radius squared.

It is sometimes puzzling to students that Poiseuille's law and the continuity rule for a stenosis (at the beginning of this section) seem contradictory. That is, one says that flow speed is less with smaller diameters (Poiseuille's law) while the other says that flow speed is greater with smaller diameters (continuity rule). How can this be so? The radius in Poiseuille's law is for the entire tube or vessel. The radius in the continuity rule is for a short portion of a vessel (the stenosis). If the radius of the entire vessel is reduced (as in vasoconstriction), flow speed is reduced. If the radius of only a short segment of a vessel is reduced (stenosis), the flow speed in the vessel is unaffected except at the stenosis where it is increased. This is because the stenosis has little effect on the flow resistance of the entire vessel if the stenosis length is small compared to the vessel length and if the lumen in the stenosis is not too small (does not approach occlusion). Figure 3.8 shows the situation for a stenosis, indicating that the overall flow resistance for the vessel is the sum of the resistances of the three parts (proximal, stenosis, distal). If the length of segment two (stenosis) is not too large and its radius is not too small, there will be a negligible effect on the overall resistance and therefore on the proximal and distal flow. However, the flow speed must increase in the stenosis to maintain continuity of volume flow. These dependencies[29] of volume flow and flow speed at the stenosis with increasing stenosis are seen in Figure 3.9.

The maximum normal flow speed in circulation is about 100 cm/s. However, in stenotic regions, flow speeds can reach a few m/s.

At the stenosis the pressure will be less than it is proximal and distal to it. This is necessary for the fluid to accelerate into the stenosis and decelerate out of it and also to maintain energy balance (pressure energy is converted to kinetic [flow] energy on entry and then vice versa on exit). This

Figure 3.9. As the diameter of the stenosis is reduced (tighter stenosis), volume flow (Q) is unaffected initially because the stenosis does not contribute substantially to the total vessel resistance. As the diameter continues to increase, the vessel resistance increases, reducing the volume flow (eventually to zero at occlusion). As the stenosis diameter decreases, flow speed increases (because of the flow continuity requirement), reaches a maximum, and then decreases to zero as the increasing flow resistance effect dominates. (Modified from Spencer MP, Reid JM: Quantitation of carotid stenosis with continuous wave (CW) doppler ultrasound. Stroke *10*(3):326–330, 1979, with permission.)

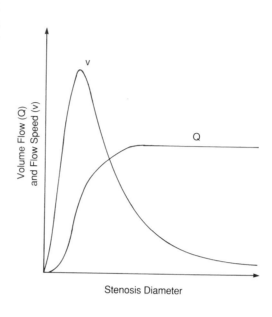

decreased pressure in regions of high flow speed is known as the bernoulli effect and is described by Bernoulli's equation, which is a description of the constant energy of the fluid flow through a stenosis ignoring viscous losses. As kinetic energy increases, pressure potential energy decreases.

$$\text{pressure} + \tfrac{1}{2} \times \text{density} \times (\text{flow speed})^2 = \text{constant energy density (energy per unit volume)}$$

Thus, the decrease in pressure that results from the increasing flow speed at the stenosis can be found from a rearrangement of Bernoulli's equation.

$$\text{pressure drop} = \tfrac{1}{2} \times \text{density} \times (\text{flow speed})^2$$
$$\Delta P = \tfrac{1}{2} \times \rho \times v^2$$

In this equation the flow speed proximal to the stenosis is assumed to be small enough to be ignored.

The disturbed flow pattern into and out of the stenosis and the increased flow speed within it can cause the onset of turbulent flow.

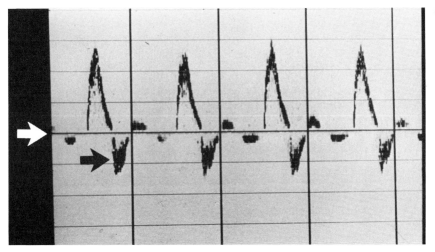

Figure 3.10. Flow reversal (negative doppler shift [black arrow] below the baseline [white arrow]) is seen in the distal abdominal aorta in diastole. (Courtesy of K. J. W. Taylor.)

Sounds produced by these disturbances and turbulence (that can be heard with a stethoscope) are called bruits. The ultimate stenosis is called an occlusion. In this case the vessel is blocked, and there is no flow.

Turbulence beyond a stenosis results in a distal pressure drop due to loss of energy (associated with pressure or flow) to heat. Doppler ultrasound is good at detecting turbulence. Spectral broadening usually indicates disturbed and turbulent flow. It will be discussed further in Chapter 6.

For calculating pressure drop across a stenotic valve or septal defect, the following equation for pressure change (pressure drop) is used in doppler echocardiography:

$$P_1 - P_2 = 4 v_2^2$$

where v_2 is the flow speed (m/s) in the jet. $P_1 - P_2$ (mm mercury) is the pressure drop across the valve or defect.

3.4
Pulsatile Flow

Previously in this chapter we considered steady flow in which pressures, flow speeds, and flow patterns (steady, disturbed, turbulent) do not change with time. This is generally the situation on the venous side of the circulatory system although cardiac pulsations and respiratory cycles can influence venous flow somewhat (for example, in the inferior vena cava). However, in arterial circulation, flow is highly pulsatile—directly experiencing the effects of the beating heart. Superimposed on the net (constant flow) are the pulsatile variations of increasing and decreasing pressure and flow speed. For steady flow, as seen in Section 3.2, volume flow is simply related to pressure difference and flow resistance. With pulsatile flow, the relationship between the varying pressure and flow rate depends upon the flow impedance, which includes the resistance formerly considered and, in addition, the inertia of the fluid as it accelerates and decelerates and the compliance (allowing expansion and contraction) of the nonrigid vessel walls. The mathematical analysis is complicated and will not be considered in detail here. Two dominant characteristics of interest in this type of flow are the windkessel effect and flow reversal. When the pressure pulse forces a fluid into a compliant vessel such as the aorta, it expands and increases the volume within it. (This is why you can feel your "pulse" on your wrist or neck.) Later in the cycle when the driving pressure is reduced, the compliant vessel can contract, producing extended flow later in the pressure cycle. This is known as the windkessel effect. In the aorta it results in continued flow in the forward direction because the aortic valve prevents flow back into the heart. In distal circulation, for example, flow into the iliac arteries, the expansion of the distendable vessels in the legs results in the reversal of flow in diastole as the pressure decreases and the distended vessels contract. Because there are no valves to prevent reverse flow here, flow reversal is observed in the iliacs and in the distal abdominal aorta (Fig. 3.10). The results, therefore, of pulsatile flow in compliant vessels include added forward flow in diastole and flow reversal in diastole, depending on location within arterial circulation. As discussed further in Chapter 6, proximal diastolic flow (absence, presence, direction, quantity) reveals much concerning the state of downstream arterioles in which flow cannot be measured.

3.5
Review

Fluids are substances that flow. Blood is a liquid that flows through the vascular system under the influence of pulsatile pressure as provided by the beating heart. Volume flow rate is proportional to pressure difference at the ends of a tube and inversely proportional to the flow resistance. The flow resistance increases with tube length and decreases (strongly) with tube diameter. Flow resistance is proportional to fluid viscosity. Five flow classifications include plug, laminar (parabolic), steady, disturbed, and turbulent. In a stenosis, flow speeds up, pressure drops, and flow is disturbed. If flow speed exceeds a critical value as described by the reynolds number, the onset of turbulence occurs. Pulsatile flow is common in arterial circulation. It results in added diastolic flow and flow reversal depending on location within the arterial system. The fluid inertia and vessel compliance are characteristics that are important in determining flow with pulsatile driving pressure.

Exercises

3.1 Which of the following are parts of the circulatory system (more than one correct answer)?
   a. heart
   b. cerebral ventricle
   c. artery
   d. arterial
   e. capillary
   f. bile duct
   g. venule
   h. vein
3.2 The _____ are the tiniest vessels in the circulatory system.
3.3 Doppler ultrasound can measure flow in (more than one correct answer).
   a. heart
   b. arteries
   c. arterioles
   d. capillaries
   e. venules
   f. veins
3.4 Which of the following are fluids?
   a. gas
   b. liquid
   c. solid
   d. a and b
   e. a, b, and c
3.5 Which of the following do (does) not flow?
   a. gas
   b. liquid
   c. solid
   d. a and b
   e. a, b, and c

3.6 To flow is to move in a _____.

3.7 Blood is made up of _____, _____, leukocytes, and platelets. Plasma is primarily _____.

3.8 A normal hematocrit is about _____ percent.
   a. 10
   b. 20
   c. 30
   d. 40
   e. 50

3.9 Which are the dominant cells in blood?
   a. erythrocytes
   b. lymphocytes
   c. monocytes
   d. leukocytes
   e. platelets

3.10 The mass per unit volume of a fluid is called its
   a. resistance
   b. viscosity
   c. kinematic viscosity
   d. impedance
   e. density

3.11 The characteristic of a fluid that offers resistance to flow is called
   a. resistance
   b. viscosity
   c. kinematic viscosity
   d. impedance
   e. density

3.12 Viscosity divided by density is called
   a. resistance
   b. viscosity
   c. kinematic viscosity
   d. impedance
   e. density

3.13 Poise is a unit of _____.

3.14 Stoke is a unit of _____.

3.15 g/mL is a unit of _____.

3.16 Give the normal values for blood of the following:
   density _____
   viscosity _____
   kinematic viscosity _____

3.17 Pressure is _____ per unit area.

3.18 Pressure is
   a. nondirectional
   b. unidirectional

    c. omnidirectional

    d. all of the above

    e. none of the above

3.19 Flow is a response to pressure _____ or _____.

3.20 If the pressure is greater at one end than it is at the other, the liquid will flow from the _____ pressure end to the _____ pressure end.

    a. higher, lower

    b. lower, higher

    c. (depends on the liquid)

    d. all of the above

    e. none of the above

3.21 A pressure difference can be generated by a _____ or by _____.

3.22 Pressure gradient is pressure _____ divided by _____ between the two pressure locations.

3.23 The flow in a tube is determined by _____ difference and _____.

3.24 If the following is increased, flow increases.

    a. pressure difference

    b. pressure gradient

    c. resistance

    d. a and b

    e. all of the above

3.25 As flow resistance increases, volume flow _____.

3.26 If pressure difference is doubled, volume flow is

    a. unchanged

    b. quartered

    c. halved

    d. doubled

    e. quadrupled

3.27 If flow resistance is doubled, volume flow is

    a. unchanged

    b. quartered

    c. halved

    d. doubled

    e. quadrupled

3.28 Tubes that carry blood in the circulatory system are called _____.

3.29 The largest vessels are

    a. arteries

    b. veins

    c. arterioles and venules

    d. capillaries

    e. a and b

3.30 The smallest vessels are

    a. arteries

    b. veins

    c. arterioles and venules

    d. capillaries

    e. a and b

3.31 Flow resistance in a vessel depends upon

    a. vessel length

    b. vessel radius

    c. blood viscosity

    d. all of the above

    e. none of the above

3.32 Flow resistance decreases with an increase in which of the following?

    a. vessel length

    b. vessel radius

    c. blood viscosity

    d. all of the above

    e. none of the above

3.33 Flow resistance depends most strongly on which of the following?

    a. vessel length

    b. vessel radius

    c. blood viscosity

    d. all of the above

    e. none of the above

3.34 Doubling the radius of a vessel decreases its resistance to _____ of the original value.

    a. one half

    b. one fourth

    c. one eighth

    d. one sixteenth

    e. one thirty-second

3.35 Volume flow decreases with an increase in which of the following?

    a. pressure difference

    b. vessel radius

    c. vessel length

    d. blood viscosity

    e. c and d

3.36 When the speed of a fluid is essentially constant across a vessel, the flow is called _____ flow.

    a. volume

    b. parabolic

    c. laminar
    d. viscous
    e. plug

3.37 _____ flow is found in larger vessels, especially in systole.
    a. volume
    b. parabolic
    c. laminar
    d. viscous
    e. plug

3.38 _____ flow is found in smaller vessels, especially in diastole.
    a. volume
    b. parabolic
    c. laminar
    d. viscous
    e. plug

3.39 _____ flow occurs when the parallel stream lines describing the flow are altered.

3.40 _____ flow involves random and chaotic flow patterns with particles flowing in all directions.

3.41 Turbulent flow occurs in a vessel when the _____ number exceeds about 2000.

3.42 A narrowing of a tube is called a _____.

3.43 Proximal to, at, and distal to a stenosis _____ must be constant.
    a. laminar flow
    b. disturbed flow
    c. turbulent flow
    d. volume flow
    e. none of the above

3.44 For the answer to Exercise 3.43 to be true, flow speed at the stenosis must be _____ that proximal and distal to it.
    a. greater than
    b. less than
    c. less turbulent than
    d. less disturbed than
    e. none of the above

3.45 Poiseuilles' equation predicts a(n) _____ in flow speed with a decrease in vessel radius.

3.46 The continuity rule predicts a(n) _____ in flow speed with a decrease in vessel diameter.

3.47 The volume flow out of the heart into the aorta is about
    a. 1 L/minute
    b. 2 L/minute
    c. 3 L/minute

d. 4 L/minute

e. 5 L/minute

3.48 The normal peak systolic flow speed out of the heart into the aorta is about

    a. 100 cm/s

    b. 200 cm/s

    c. 300 cm/s

    d. 400 cm/s

    e. 500 cm/s

3.49 In a stenosis the pressure is _____ the proximal and distal values.

    a. less than

    b. equal to

    c. greater than

    d. (depends on the fluid)

    e. none of the above

3.50 Added forward flow and flow reversal in diastole are results of _____ flow.

    a. volume

    b. turbulent

    c. laminar

    d. disturbed

    e. pulsatile

3.51 Calculate the flow speed above which turbulent blood flow should occur in the aorta. Assume a diameter of 2 cm and 2000 for the reynolds number.

3.52 For the stenosis shown in Figure 3.8, d_1 = 2 cm, d_2 = 1 cm, and d_3 = 2 cm. For 50 mL/s blood flowing through the stenosis, find the flow speeds and the reynolds numbers proximal to, at, and distal to the stenosis.

3.53 Turbulence generally occurs when reynolds numbers exceed

    a. 100

    b. 200

    c. 1000

    d. 2000

    e. a and b

3.54 As stenosis diameter decreases, the following pass(es) through a maximum.

    a. flow speed at the stenosis

    b. flow speed proximal to stenosis

    c. volume flow

    d. doppler shift at the stenosis

    e. a and d

Chapter 4

Doppler Effect

The doppler effect is a change in frequency or wavelength due to motion of the wave source, receiver, or a reflector of the wave. If the source is moving toward the receiver, the receiver is moving toward the source, or the reflector is moving toward the source and receiver, the received wave will have a higher frequency than would be experienced without the motion. Conversely, if the motion is away (receding), the received wave will have a lower frequency. The amount of increase or decrease in the frequency depends upon the speed of motion, the angle between the wave direction and the motion direction, and the frequency of the wave emitted by the source. These aspects of the doppler effect will be treated separately in the sections of this chapter.

4.1
Doppler Effect

The doppler effect occurs for any kind of wave but is commonly experienced in life with sound. This is because speeds of motion experienced commonly can be a significant fraction of the speed of sound (a few percent). With light this is not true and only astronomical motions provide speeds great enough to produce a readily observable doppler effect. This will be discussed further in the next section.

A qualitative description of the doppler effect is presented in the introductory paragraph to this chapter. A quantitative description of the doppler effect is provided by the doppler equation. It can be derived for the three situations previously mentioned, as follows:

For a moving receiver (Fig. 4.1) approaching the source, more cycles of the wave will be encountered in a second than would be if the receiver were stationary. The speed of receiver motion divided by the wavelength yields the increase in the number of cycles encountered per second (the increase in received frequency). The change in frequency due to motion is called the doppler shift. In this case it is positive, that is, the received frequency will be greater than that without the motion.

received frequency

$$= \text{emitted frequency} \left[\frac{\text{propagation speed} + \text{receiver speed}}{\text{propagation speed}} \right]$$

$$f_r = f_o \left[\frac{c + v_r}{c} \right]$$

If the receiver approaches the source at the speed of sound, the received frequency will be twice the source frequency and the doppler shift is equal

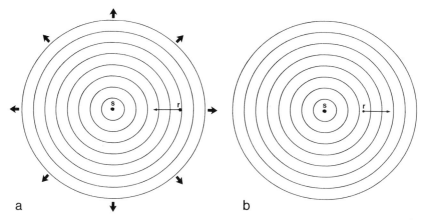

a   b

Figure 4.1. (a) A receiver (r) moving toward the source (s) experiences a higher frequency (more cycles per second) than a stationary one would. (b) A receiver moving away from the source experiences a lower frequency than a stationary one would.

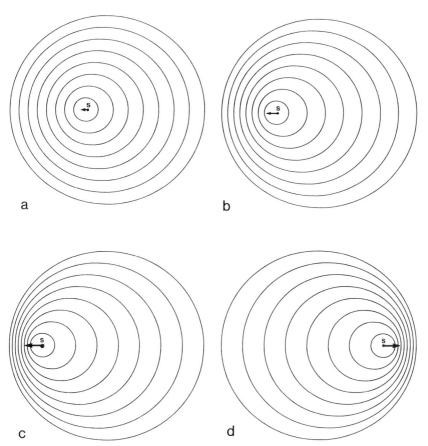

Figure 4.2. A moving source (s) of sound produces a shorter wavelength (higher frequency) ahead of it and a longer wavelength (lower frequency) behind it compared to the wavelengths at the sides, which are the same as for a stationary source: (a) slow speed; (b) medium speed; (c) high speed; (d) movement in opposite direction.

to the source frequency. If the receiver moves away from the source, the above equations are the same except a minus sign appears in place of the plus. For a receiver moving away from the source at the speed of the wave, no cycles are experienced by the receiver and the received frequency is zero. In this case the (negative) doppler shift is equal to the source frequency.

For a moving source and a stationary receiver, the cycles are compressed in front of the source moving into the wave (Fig. 4.2). The emitted wavelength with this source motion is as follows:

emitted wavelength

$$= \text{source wavelength} \left[\frac{\text{propagation speed} - \text{source speed}}{\text{propagation speed}} \right]$$

$$\lambda_e = \lambda_o \left[\frac{c - v_s}{c} \right]$$

The source wavelength is the wavelength that would be observed in the traveling wave without source motion. The source motion causes wave compression or shortening of the wavelength ahead of it. This decreased wavelength results in an increased frequency observed by a stationary receiver in front of the approaching source.

emitted frequency

$$= \text{source frequency} \left[\frac{\text{propagation speed}}{\text{propagation speed} - \text{source speed}} \right]$$

$$f_e = f_o \left[\frac{c}{c - v_s} \right]$$

If the source speed approaches the wave speed, the emitted frequency approaches infinity. This is known as a shock wave, an example of which is the sonic boom received from aircraft traveling at or beyond the speed of sound. For motion away from the receiver, the previous equation applies except that the minus sign is replaced by a plus sign. For a source speed equal to the wave speed away from the receiver, the emitted frequency is equal to one half the source frequency.

A moving reflector (Fig. 4.3) or a scatterer of a wave is a combination of both a moving receiver and emitter. It is described by a combination of the two doppler equations presented above. The source frequency of the scatterer is equal to that which it receives so that its emitted frequency is as follows:

emitted frequency

$$= \text{source frequency} \left[\frac{\text{propagation speed} + \text{scatterer speed}}{\text{propagation speed} - \text{scatterer speed}} \right]$$

$$f_e = f_o \left[\frac{c + v}{c - v} \right]$$

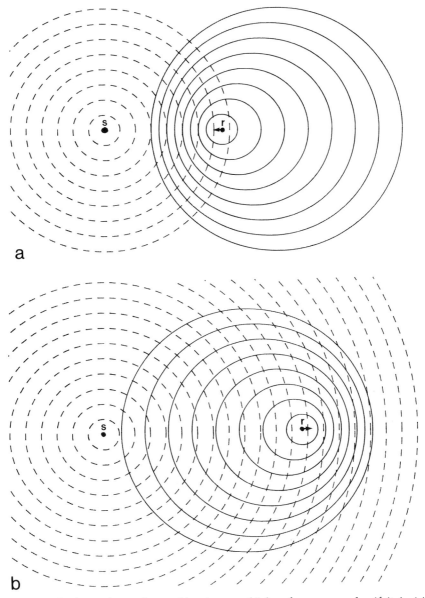

Figure 4.3. A moving reflector (r) returns a higher frequency echo if it is (a) approaching the source (s) and receiver (s) or a lower frequency echo if it is (b) moving away from the source and receiver.

As an example, let the source frequency be 5 MHz, the scatterer speed be 50 cm/s, and the wave (sound) speed be 1540 m/s. The frequency emitted by the approaching scatterer and thus received by the receiver is as follows:

$$f_e = 5 \left[\frac{1540 + 0.5}{1540 - 0.5} \right] = 5.0032$$

The received frequency is greater than the source frequency with a positive doppler shift of 0.0032 MHz or 3.2 kHz. For a scatterer moving away from a receiver, the signs in the equation are reversed (minus in numerator, plus in denominator). Other examples using various source frequencies and scatterer speeds are included elsewhere in this chapter.

The doppler shift for a moving scatterer is equal to the emitted (and received) frequency derived above minus the source frequency.

doppler shift = emitted frequency − source frequency

$$= \text{source frequency} \left[\frac{2 \times \text{scatterer speed}}{\text{propagation speed} - \text{scatterer speed}} \right]$$

$$f_D = f_e - f_o$$

$$= f_o \left[\frac{2v}{c - v} \right]$$

The factor of two in the doppler equation, then, is a result of two doppler shifts for a scatterer: (1) the doppler shift as a moving receiver encounters the wave and (2) the doppler shift as the moving emitter reradiates the wave. Another way to view the two factors is considering the transducer to be the source and receiver of sound separated by the round-trip sound path distance that is twice the distance from transducer to reflector. As the reflector approaches or recedes from the transducer, this (round-trip) distance is reduced at a rate double the speed of the reflector (see Exercises 4.51 and 4.52).

Physiologic blood flow speeds, even in extreme cases, are no more than a few percent of the speed of sound in tissues (1540 m/s). Because flow speed is small compared to sound speed, it may be ignored in the denominator, yielding the form shown in Figure 4.4 where the effect of doppler angle (Section 4.3) is included. Because propagation speed divided by frequency is equal to wavelength, the following form of the doppler equation is valid.

$$f_D = \frac{2 f v \cos \theta}{c}$$

$$v = \frac{f_D c}{2 f \cos \theta}$$

Figure 4.4. The three basic doppler equations for a reflector or scatterer of sound.

$$v \; (cm/s) = \frac{77 \; f_D \; (kHz)}{f \; (MHz) \cos \theta}$$

$$\text{doppler shift} = \frac{2 \times \text{scatterer speed}}{\text{wavelength}} \qquad f_D = \frac{2v}{\lambda}$$

The doppler shift for a moving receiver is as follows:

$$\text{doppler shift} = \text{source frequency} \left[\frac{\text{receiver speed}}{\text{propagation speed}} \right]$$

$$f_D = f_o \left[\frac{v_r}{c} \right]$$

The doppler shift for a moving emitter is as follows:

$$\text{doppler shift} = \text{source frequency} \left[\frac{\text{source speed}}{\text{propagation speed} - \text{source speed}} \right]$$

$$f_D = f_o \left[\frac{v_s}{c - v_s} \right]$$

The doppler shift for the case of a moving receiver is not the same as that for a moving emitter with the same speed of motion (see Exercise 4.41).

However, there is a negligible difference between the two for low speeds (compared to the speed of sound).

The doppler shift for a moving scatterer is summarized in symbolic form in Figure 4.4 where the scatterer speed has been eliminated in the denominator and doppler angle has been included. These two aspects will be discussed later in this chapter. It is the doppler shift that the instruments described in Chapter 5 detect. However, it is the speed of motion or flow of blood in which we are normally interested. The doppler equation can be rearranged to place the speed of motion alone on the left side of the equation as follows (see Fig. 4.4):

$$\text{scatterer speed} = \left[\frac{\text{doppler shift} \times \text{propagation speed}}{2 \times \text{source frequency} \times \text{cosine doppler angle}} \right]$$

$$v = \left[\frac{f_D c}{2f \cos \theta_D} \right]$$

Substituting in the speed of sound and using units as indicated for the various quantities yields the equation in the following form (see Fig. 4.4):

$$\text{scatterer speed (cm/s)} = \left[\frac{77 \times \text{doppler shift (kHz)}}{\text{source frequency (MHz)} \times \text{cosine doppler angle}} \right]$$

$$v = \left[\frac{77 \times f_D}{f \times \cos \theta_D} \right]$$

The speed of sound used here is the average speed of sound in soft tissues—1540 m/s or 1.54 mm/μs. It is tempting to use the speed of sound in blood,[30,31] 1570–1575 m/s. However, this may not be appropriate when considering the interesting clarification given in the next paragraph.

There is a complication in the consideration of the doppler effect for ultrasound scattered by cells in circulating blood that has not been considered in the previous discussion. The cells that scatter the ultrasound move along with the surrounding medium (plasma) rather than moving through it as is the case for an ambulance moving through air (the common illustration of the doppler effect with the approaching siren). The fact that the scatterers are moving along with the medium means that the doppler effect does not occur at the scatterer boundary (the boundary between the cell and plasma). Nevertheless, the doppler effect is observed when an ultrasound beam interacts with flowing blood. In fact, the doppler effect occurs at the boundary between the stationary tissue (the internal vessel wall or intima) and the blood. As the sound crosses this boundary, it encounters a moving propagation medium (blood plasma) with the result that the wavelength is decreased if the blood is flowing toward the transducer or increased if it is flowing away (Fig. 4.5). In other words, the doppler shift occurs at the vessel wall and not at the cell membrane.[32-34] The doppler shift is doubled as with the previous consideration of a moving scatterer because as the reradiated (scattered) wave exits the moving blood and enters the stationary tissue there is a second positive doppler shift (or a second negative doppler shift if the flow is away from the transducer) (see Fig. 4.5). This is the most accurate explanation for the factor of two in the doppler equation.

4.2
Speed

The doppler equation indicates that the doppler shift is proportional to the speed of the moving object (source, receiver, or scatterer) and, more specifically, it is proportional to the ratio of that speed to the wave propagation speed. This is why, as mentioned in Section 4.1, the doppler effect with light is not normally experienced in life while, with sound, it is. The speed of light is about 1 million times that of sound (see Table 2.1).

The fact that the doppler shift is proportional to the scatterer speed and, therefore, to blood flow speed explains why the doppler effect is so useful in medical diagnosis. The doppler instruments measure the doppler shift. It is the blood flow in which we are interested. The measured shifts are proportional to flow speed, knowledge of which we desire.

If a yellow automobile could travel at 100 million miles per hour (15 percent the speed of light), the positive doppler shift as it approached would cause it to appear blue, there would be a flash of yellow as it passed by, and then it would appear to be a red vehicle as it receded owing to the doppler downshift (see Color Plate I). Fifteen percent of the speed of sound in air is 110 miles per hour. If a vehicle approached at this speed emitting a tone of 262 Hz (middle C), the tone heard by a stationary observer would be 308 Hz (D = 294 Hz) and the tone heard after the vehicle passed and was receding would be 223 Hz (A = 220 Hz). Our human auditory system is capable of detecting changes much smaller than this so that we can hear the doppler shift occur as a sound-emitting vehicle passes at much lower speeds. The doppler shift with light has been useful

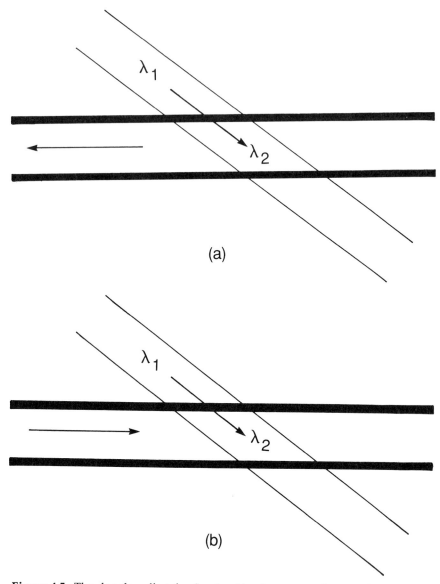

Figure 4.5. The doppler effect for flowing blood occurs at the vessel wall-blood boundary. (a) As the sound crosses the vessel into approaching blood, the wavelength is shortened. (b) As the sound crosses the vessel into receding blood, the wavelength is lengthened.

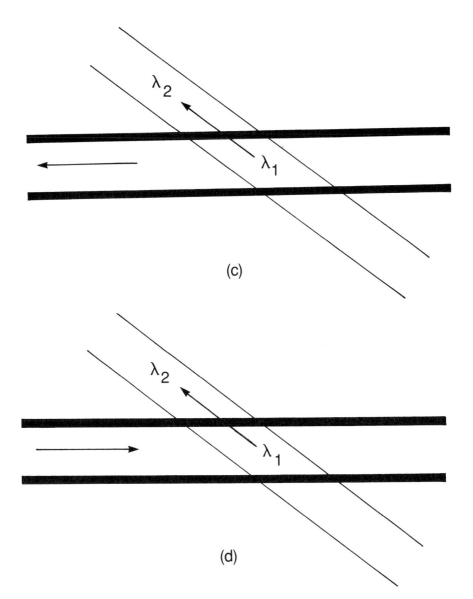

Figure 4.5 *Continued* (c) As sound exits approaching blood, the wavelength is shortened. (d) As sound exits receding blood, the wavelength is lengthened.

in determining motion of light emitting stars and galaxies in the universe. These all have red shifts indicating motion away from us. Furthermore, the red shifts and calculated speeds of motion are proportional to the distances of the objects. This indicates that the universe is expanding and had its origin at a common location at some point in time long past. More detailed motions of nearer objects such as our sun have been made possible by doppler shift measurements of the light from various points located on them.

Using electromagnetic microwaves, doppler radar has been applied in weather forecasting and aviation safety. It is also used in the familiar application of police radar detection of vehicle speeds on highways. This is an example of a detected doppler shift resulting from reflection from a moving object.

Ultrasonic burglar alarms and door openers are quite common in homes and public buildings. These also use the doppler shift resulting from a moving reflector (person in motion). These systems operate around 25 kHz, emitting ultrasound into and receiving it from the air. A person walking at one step per second generates a doppler shift of about 65 Hz in such a system.[35]

With diagnostic medical ultrasound, stationary transducers are used to emit and receive the ultrasound. The doppler effect is a result of the motion of blood, the flow of which we wish to measure.

Another long-standing application of doppler ultrasound in medicine is in monitoring fetal heartbeat during labor and delivery. Instruments that perform this function can be less sophisticated and less sensitive than blood flow measurement systems because the echoes from the beating heart are much stronger than those coming from blood. Doppler shifts resulting from various typical physiologic flow speeds are given in Table 4.1. Figure 4.6 illustrates the proportional dependence of doppler shift on

Table 4.1
Doppler Frequency Shifts for Various Scatterer Speeds Toward the Sound Source*

Incident Frequency (MHz)	Scatterer Speed (cm/s)	Reflected Frequency (MHz)	Doppler Shift (kHz)
2	50	2.0013	1.3
5	50	5.0032	3.2
10	50	10.0065	6.5
2	200	2.0052	5.2
5	200	5.013	13.0
10	200	10.026	26.0

*Motion away from the source would yield negative doppler shifts.

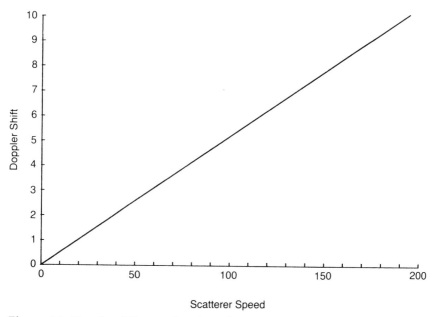

Figure 4.6. Doppler shift as a function of scatterer speed as determined by the doppler equation. (From Kremkau FW: Seeing and hearing blood flow noninvasively using the doppler shift. Diagn Imaging 7:131, 1985. Reprinted with permission.)

scatterer speed. The primary effect of a change in blood flow speed is a change in doppler shift. The strength, intensity, or power of the returning doppler-shifted echoes is not affected by the flow speed. Such an effect is not predicted by the doppler equation and has not been found in experimental investigations.[36]

The minimum detectable blood flow speed with doppler ultrasound (color-flow instruments—Section 5.4) is a few mm/s. The maximum is determined by aliasing (Section 7.1) with pulsed doppler instruments (Section 5.2). In principle, there is no upper limit for continuous-wave instruments (Section 5.1). The range of commonly detected normal flow speeds is 10 to 100 cm/s.

4.3
Angle

If the direction of sound propagation is directly opposite to the flow direction, the maximum positive doppler shift is obtained. If the flow speed and propagation speed directions are the same (parallel), the maximum negative doppler shift is obtained. If the angle between these two directions (Fig. 4.7) is nonzero, lesser doppler shifts will occur. As seen in the doppler equation (see Fig. 4.4), the dependence on the doppler angle is in the form of a cosine. Table 4.2 gives cosine values for various angles.

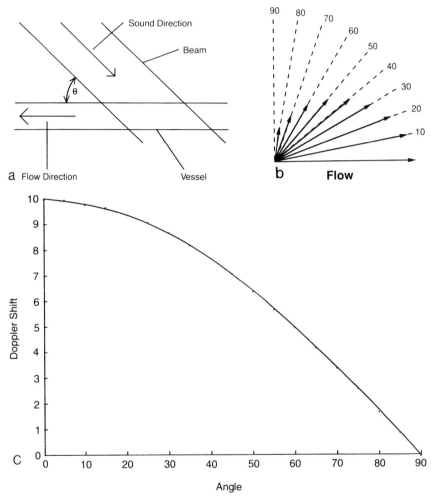

Figure 4.7. (a) Angle θ is the angle between the direction of flow and the sound propagation direction. (From Kremkau FW: Technical considerations, equipment, and physics of duplex sonography. *In* Grant EG, White EM: Duplex Sonography. New York, Springer-Verlag, 1988. Reprinted with permission.) (b) As doppler angle increases, echo doppler shift frequency decreases. (c) Doppler shift as a function of angle as determined by the doppler equation. (From Kremkau FW: Seeing and hearing blood flow noninvasively using the doppler shift. Diagn Imaging 7:131, 1985. Reprinted with permission.)

Table 4.2
Cosines for Various Angles

Angle A (Degrees)	cos A
0	1.00
5	0.996
10	0.98
15	0.97
20	0.94
25	0.91
30	0.87
35	0.82
40	0.77
45	0.71
50	0.64
55	0.57
60	0.50
65	0.42
70	0.34
75	0.26
80	0.17
85	0.09
90	0.00

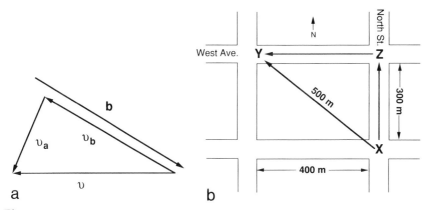

Figure 4.8. (a) The flow velocity vector (v) can be broken up into two components, one (v_b) that is parallel to the sound beam direction (b) and one (v_a) that is perpendicular to the sound beam direction. (b) An analogy to the vector components in (a) using a city block example. To get from X to Y one could walk diagonally across the block, a distance of 500 meters. However, if buildings prevented that path, an alternate route would be 300 meters north on North Street and then 400 meters west on West Avenue. The 500 meter northwest vector from X to Y is equivalent to a 300 meter north vector plus a 400 meter west vector (i.e., the result is the same—depart from X and arrive at Y). In this example, the component of the XY vector parallel to North Street is the XZ vector and the component parallel to West Avenue is the ZY vector.

Table 4.3
Doppler Frequency Shifts for Various
Angles and Scatterer Speeds Toward
the Sound Source of Frequency 5 MHz

Scatterer Speed (cm/s)	Angle (°)	Doppler Shift (kHz)
100	0	6.5
100	30	5.6
100	60	3.2
100	90	0.0
300	0	19.0
300	30	17.0
300	60	9.7
300	90	0.0

For angles greater than 90 degrees, the cosine is negative, yielding the negative doppler shift we expect since flow is receding in that case. The cosine gives the component of the flow velocity vector that is parallel to the sound beam (Fig. 4.8). For a given flow, the greater the doppler angle, the less the doppler shift (Fig. 4.7b,c). Examples of doppler shifts for various angles are listed in Table 4.3.

It is extremely important to realize that the flow speed calculations based on doppler shift measurements can only be done with a knowledge of the doppler angle involved. They, therefore, are only as good as the accuracy of the estimate or measurement of that angle. Measurement is normally done by orienting a line on the anatomic display such that it is parallel to the presumed direction of flow (usually parallel to vessel walls). This is a subjective operation performed by the sonographer. Error in this estimation of the doppler angle is more critical at large angles than it is at

Table 4.4
Percent Error for 2- and 5-Degree Angle Errors

True Angle (Degrees)	Percent Error for 2-Degree Error	Percent Error for 5-Degree Error
0	0.06	0.38
10	0.68	1.9
20	1.3	3.6
30	2.0	5.4
40	3.0	7.7
50	3.9	9.1
60	5.6	12
70	8.7	19
80	16	33

small ones. Table 4.4 gives error values for various angles. Figure 4.9 shows how the error in calculated flow speed increases with angle for a 5-degree angle measurement error. For this reason, and because doppler shifts become very small at large angles, reducing the system sensitivity, doppler measurements (and particularly calculated flow speeds) are not reliably achieved at doppler angles greater than about 60 to 70 degrees. Because normally the ultrasound beam does not travel directly down the vessel (because the transducer is offset from the vessel axis—see Fig. 4.6), the doppler angle is dependent upon the direction in which the beam is pointed. In principle, if everything is done correctly, the calculated flow speed in the vessel should be the same regardless of the doppler angle. That is, if the vessel is straight and of uniform diameter and has uniform flow within it, the same flow speed should be found no matter how (at

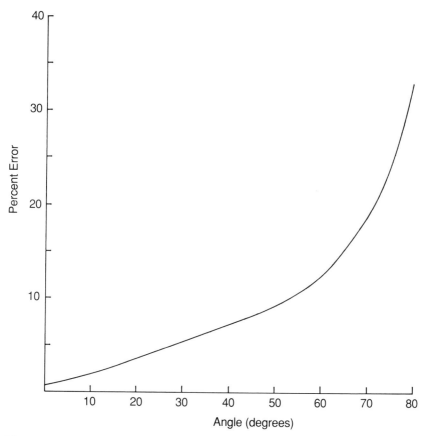

Figure 4.9. Percent cosine error versus doppler angle for a 5-degree angle error.

Table 4.5
Doppler Shifts (for 4 MHz) at Various
Doppler Angles for the Same Flow
Ideally Yield a Consistent Calculated
Flow Speed

Doppler Shift (kHz)	Angle (Degrees)	Calculated Flow Speed (cm/s)
2.25	30	50
1.99	40	50
1.84	45	50
1.67	50	50
1.30	60	50

what angle) the beam intersects the vessel (Table 4.5). Since this is commonly not found to be the case, inaccuracies in angle estimation are probably being observed. Also, flow is probably not uniform even in unobstructed vessels.[26,37–39] Examples of correct and incorrect handling of doppler angle are shown in Figure 5.12.

Because sound propagation speed is not the same in blood as it is in soft tissues (it is slightly greater in blood), refraction occurs as the sound crosses the boundary from the vessel wall into the blood. This introduces an error in the estimated angle, particularly for small doppler angles. However, the error in the cosine of the angle appears to be only around 2 percent. It is important to know that a critical angle is reached at about 25 degrees where the sound no longer enters the blood at all but is totally reflected at the wall-blood boundary. The increase in reflected intensity (and therefore decrease in transmitted intensity) at this boundary with decreasing doppler angle causes the effectiveness of doppler measurements to be reduced at doppler angles less than about 30 degrees. However, in doppler echocardiography doppler angles of nearly zero are achieved and zero is commonly assumed (i.e., angle correction is not attempted as it is in vascular work).

Because the doppler measurement is angle dependent (that is, the doppler method only measures the component of the flow vector that is parallel to the sound beam), a single doppler measurement can correspond to many different flow velocities (speeds and directions) (Fig. 4.10). If two measurements of the same flow are made at two different angles, the correct flow speed and direction (velocity) can be obtained.

Color Plate VIa gives a color-flow example of no doppler shift that could be interpreted as an occluded vessel. However, a 90-degree doppler angle is the cause. When a different angle is achieved, flow (color) appears in the vessel (see Color Plate VIb).

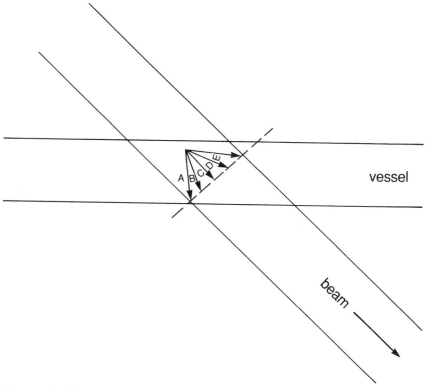

Figure 4.10. Flow velocity vectors A, B, C, D, and E each have the same component along the beam axis (therefore yield the same doppler shift frequency). (Modified from Phillips DJ, Beach KW, Primozich J, Strandness DE: Should results of ultrasound doppler studies be reported in units of frequency or velocity? Ultrasound Med Biol 15:205–212, 1989, with permission.)

The primary effect of a change in doppler angle is a change in doppler shift. The strength, intensity, or power of the returning doppler-shifted echoes is not affected by angle.

In conclusion, it must be emphasized that to proceed from a measurement of doppler shift frequency to a calculation of flow speed, doppler angle must be known or correctly assumed. Otherwise, an incorrect flow speed calculation will result.

We have only considered in this discussion the doppler angle in the scan plane. It must be remembered that the vessel may not be parallel to the imaging scan plane, which includes the doppler beam, so that there may be a component of doppler angle between the flow direction and the scan plane. Thus, the three-dimensional character of the components involved in the process (vessel anatomy, flow, and ultrasound image) must be kept in mind.

4.4
Frequency

For a given flow in a vessel, the doppler shift measured by an instrument is proportional (Fig. 4.11) to the operating frequency of the instrument. Table 4.1 gives doppler shifts for various frequencies. Thus, measurement of doppler shifts from flow in the same vessel using two different instruments operating at 2 MHz and 4 MHz will yield two different doppler shifts with the higher frequency instrument having a doppler shift double that of the lower frequency instrument. When comparing doppler shifts, therefore, frequency of the devices must be accounted for. In the calculation of flow speed, the operating frequency is incorporated. Thus, comparisons of flow speeds between different instru-

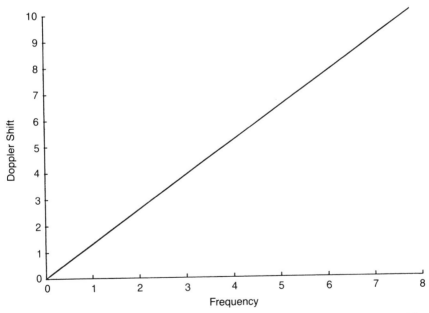

Figure 4.11. Doppler shift as a function of operating frequency as determined by the doppler equation. (From Kremkau FW: Seeing and hearing blood flow noninvasively using the doppler shift. Diagn Imaging 7:131, 1985. Reprinted with permission.)

ments have taken into account this variable. However, recall that such calculations depend upon the accuracy of the angle estimation. When the angle is unknown and doppler shift data are used, the ratio of the doppler shift to the operating frequency facilitates comparisons between different instruments because it has the same value for a given flow and angle regardless of operating frequency.[40] Although angle affects the measurement, this index does eliminate one variable in the comparisons and brings us one step closer to a uniform comparison index. For a flow speed of 1 m/s and an angle of 45 degrees, this index is approximately equal to 1 kHz/MHz.

Thus far, we have assumed that for a given frequency ultrasound beam, the only thing that produces a frequency shift in the returning echoes is the motion associated with blood flow. In truth, other factors produce a frequency shift also, four of which will be mentioned here. Erythrocytes are small compared to the wavelengths of ultrasound used. The echo intensity from such small objects is proportional to frequency to the fourth power. Because ultrasound pulses involve a range of frequencies (described by the band width), the higher frequencies are scattered more strongly while the lower are scattered less strongly. This produces a positive frequency shift (not a doppler shift) in the returning echoes. In contrast, attenuation of ultrasound in tissues increases with frequency. Therefore, as the sound travels out and the echoes travel back, the higher frequencies within the band width are attenuated more than the lower ones. This causes a downshift in the mean frequency of the returning echoes. Nonlinear characteristics of the tissue as a sound propagation medium cause higher harmonic frequencies to be generated as the sound wave converts from a sinusoidal form to a sawtooth form. This produces an increase in the mean frequency of the sound as it travels. Finally, electrical properties of the transducer cause it to treat various frequencies more or less efficiently than others. This can result in an increase or decrease in the mean frequency. The net result of these up- and downshifts is almost impossible to predict but, apparently, has a negligible effect on the doppler shifts encountered physiologically.

The frequency dependencies of scattering and attenuation mentioned in the previous paragraph compete in the sense that scattering characteristics produce stronger echoes with higher frequencies while the attenuation reduces the strength of higher frequency echoes received at the transducer. The attenuation has the dominant effect so that higher frequencies do not penetrate as effectively as lower ones. Taking both into account, a practical rule is that the optimum ultrasound frequency to use for measurements at a given depth is approximately equal to 90 divided by the depth in millimeters.[13] This yields the optimum operating frequency in megahertz. In practice, frequencies comparable to that used for sonography are used for doppler measurements (that is, 2 to 10 MHz). Doppler frequencies for given depth applications are, in practice, slightly less than for imaging at that depth.

4.5
Review

The doppler effect is a change in frequency or wavelength resulting from motion. In medical ultrasound applications the motion is either that

Table 4.6
Doppler Shifts for Various Frequencies, Angles, and Speeds

Frequency (MHz)	Angle (Degrees)	Speed (cm/s)	Shift (kHz)
2	0	10	0.26
2	0	50	1.30
2	0	100	2.60
2	30	10	0.22
2	30	50	1.12
2	30	100	2.25
2	45	10	0.18
2	45	50	0.92
2	45	100	1.84
2	60	10	0.13
2	60	50	0.65
2	60	100	1.30
5	0	10	0.65
5	0	50	3.25
5	0	100	6.49
5	30	10	0.56
5	30	50	2.81
5	30	100	5.62
5	45	10	0.46
5	45	50	2.30
5	45	100	4.59
5	60	10	0.32
5	60	50	1.62
5	60	100	3.25
10	0	10	1.30
10	0	50	6.49
10	0	100	13.0
10	30	10	1.12
10	30	50	5.62
10	30	100	11.2
10	45	10	0.92
10	45	50	4.59
10	45	100	9.18
10	60	10	0.65
10	60	50	3.25
10	60	100	6.49

of the heart or blood flow in circulation. The change in frequency of the returning echoes with respect to the emitted frequency is called the doppler shift. For flow toward the transducer, it is positive; for flow away, it is negative. The doppler shift depends upon the speed of the scatterers of sound, the angle between their direction and that of the sound propagation, and the operating frequency of the doppler system. Thus, reporting a doppler shift frequency without specifying the operating frequency and doppler angle is incomplete. A moving scatterer of sound produces a double doppler shift. Greater flow speeds and smaller doppler angles produce larger doppler shifts but not stronger echoes. Higher operating frequencies produce larger doppler shifts. Typical ranges of flow speeds (10 to 100 cm/s), doppler angles (30 to 60 degrees), and operating frequencies (2 to 10 MHz) yield doppler shifts in the range 100 Hz to 11 kHz for vascular studies. In doppler echocardiography where zero angle and speeds of a few meters per second can be encountered, doppler shifts can be as high as 30 kHz. Table 4.6 gives doppler shifts for various frequencies, angles, and speeds.

Exercises

4.1 The _____ effect is used to detect and measure _____ in vessels.

4.2 Motion of an echo-generating structure causes an echo to have a different _____ than the emitted pulse.

4.3 The doppler effect is a change in reflected _____ caused by reflector _____.

4.4 If the reflector is moving toward the source, the reflected frequency is _____ than the incident frequency.

4.5 If the reflector is moving away from the source, the reflected frequency is _____ than the incident frequency.

4.6 If the reflector is stationary with respect to the source, the reflected frequency is _____ _____ the incident frequency.

4.7 Measurement of doppler shift yields information about reflector _____.

4.8 If the incident frequency is 1 MHz, the propagation speed is 1600 m/s, and the reflector speed is 16 m/s toward the source, the doppler shift is _____ MHz, and the reflected frequency is _____ MHz.

4.9 If 2-MHz ultrasound is reflected from a soft tissue boundary moving at 10 m/s toward the source, the doppler shift is _____ MHz.

4.10 If 2-MHz ultrasound is reflected from a soft tissue boundary moving at 10 m/s away from the source, the doppler shift is _____ MHz.

4.11 Doppler shift is the difference between _____ and
_____ frequencies.

4.12 When incident sound direction and reflector motion are not parallel,
calculation of the reflected frequency involves the _____
of the angle between these directions.

4.13 If the angle between incident sound direction and reflector motion is
60 degrees, the doppler shift and reflected frequency in Exercise 4.8
are _____ MHz and _____ MHz.

4.14 If the angle between incident sound direction and reflector motion is
90 degrees, the cosine of the angle is _____, and the reflected frequency in Exercise 4.8 is _____ MHz.

4.15 A policeman in a (doppler) radar-equipped patrol car detects the
speed of an automobile to be 55 mph. If the angle between the radar
beam and the direction of the automobile is 60 degrees, the actual
speed of the automobile is _____ mph.

4.16 Fill in the missing values in the table.

f (MHz)	v (cm/s)	θ (Degrees)	f_D (kHz)
2.5	50	0	(a)
5	50	(b)	3.25
7.5	(c)	0	4.87
(d)	100	0	3.25
5	100	0	(e)
7.5	100	(f)	9.74
2.5	(g)	0	4.87
(h)	150	0	9.74
7.5	150	0	(i)
5	50	30	(j)
5	50	(k)	1.62
5	50	(l)	0
5	(m)	30	5.62
5	100	60	(n)
5	(o)	90	0
5	150	(p)	8.44
(q)	150	60	4.87
5	150	90	(r)

4.17 The maximum normal flow speed encountered in the circulatory system is approximately

    a. 1 mm/s
    b. 1 cm/s
    c. 100 cm/s
    d. 100 m/s
    e. 1 km/s

4.18 For operating frequency 2 MHz, flow speed 10 cm/s, and doppler angle 0, calculate the doppler shift.

4.19 For operating frequency 4 MHz, flow speed 10 cm/s, and doppler angle 30 degrees, calculate the doppler shift.

4.20 For operating frequency 6 MHz, flow speed 50 cm/s, and doppler angle 60 degrees, calculate the doppler shift.

4.21 For operating frequency 5 MHz, doppler angle 45 degrees, and doppler shift 4.60 kHz, calculate the flow speed.

4.22 For operating frequency 6 MHz, doppler angle 60 degrees, and doppler shift 1.95 kHz, calculate the flow speed.

4.23 If the propagation speed in blood is greater than that in the surrounding tissue, the effect of refraction is to (increase or decrease?) the doppler angle.

4.24 The result in Exercise 4.23 (increases or decreases?) the doppler shift frequency.

4.25 What is the doppler shift if a receiver is moving toward a 5-MHz source at the speed of sound?

4.26 If a receiver is moving away from a 5-MHz source at the speed of sound, what is the doppler shift?

4.27 In Exercise 4.26, what frequency does the receiver detect?

4.28 If a 5-MHz source moves toward a receiver at the speed of sound, what frequency is received?

4.29 If a 5-MHz source moves away from a receiver at the speed of sound, what frequency is received?

4.30 The doppler shifts for a moving source, a moving receiver, and a moving reflector (all moving at the same speed) produce the same doppler shifts. True or false?

4.31 For blood flowing in a vessel, where does the doppler shift occur?

4.32 In view of the answer to Exercise 4.31, are blood cells necessary for utilizing doppler ultrasound? Why or why not?

4.33 Physiologic flow speeds can be as much as _____ percent of the propagation speed in soft tissues.
    a. 0.01
    b. 0.3
    c. 5
    d. 10
    e. 50

4.34 Which doppler angle gives the greatest doppler shift?

    a. −90
    b. −45
    c. 0
    d. 45
    e. 90

4.35 To proceed from a measurement of doppler shift frequency to a calculation of flow speed, _____ _____ must be known or correctly assumed.

4.36 The intensity of returning doppler-shifted echoes is not affected by _____ or _____.

4.37 Doppler shift frequency is not dependent on
    a. amplitude
    b. flow speed
    c. operating frequency
    d. doppler angle
    e. propagation speed

4.38 If operating frequency is doubled, doppler shift is _____.

4.39 If flow speed is doubled, doppler shift is _____.

4.40 If doppler angle is increased, doppler shift is _____.

4.41 Calculate the 5-MHz doppler shifts (a) for a receiver moving at 100 m/s, (b) for a source moving at 100 m/s, and (c) for a reflector moving at 100 m/s.

4.42 In Figure 4.6, what is the operating frequency, assuming shift in kHz, speed in cm/s, and 0 doppler angle? Assuming a 60-degree angle?

4.43 In Figure 4.11, what is scatterer speed, assuming frequency in MHz and a 0 doppler angle? Assuming a 60-degree angle?

4.44 In Figure 4.7c, what is the operating frequency, assuming angle in degrees and 100 cm/s scatterer speed?

4.45 In Figure 4.7c, what is scatterer speed assuming angle in degrees and 5 MHz operating frequency?

4.46 For doppler angle 60 degrees, flow speed 1.5 m/s, and operating frequency 5 MHz, the doppler shift is _____ kHz, which is _____ percent of the operating frequency.

4.47 In Figure 4.12, which angle is the incidence angle? Which angle is the doppler angle? Is this true if refraction occurs? Which angle is the transmission angle? If there is no refraction, which two angles are equal? Incidence angle plus doppler angle (no refraction) equals what?

4.48 The cosine of an angle can be no greater than
    a. 10
    b. 1
    c. 0
    d. −1
    e. −10

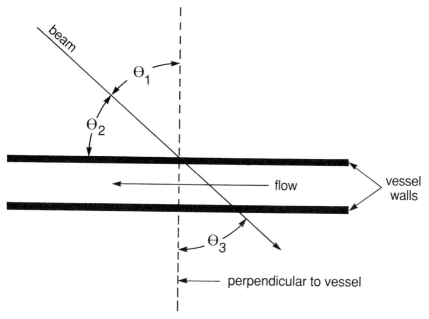

Figure 4.12. Angles for Exercise 4.47.

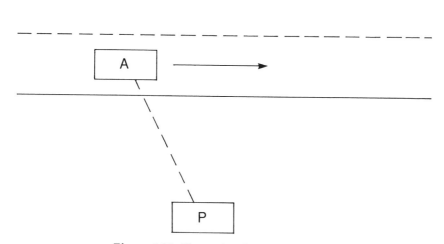

Figure 4.13. Illustration for Exercise 4.54.

4.49 The cosine of an angle can be no less than
  a. 10
  b. 1
  c. 0
  d. −1
  e. −10

4.50 The difference between the doppler shift for a moving receiver and a moving source is negligible if the speed is _____ enough.

4.51 As a reflector approaches a transducer at 50 cm/s, the round-trip distance between them is reduced at the rate _____ cm/s.

4.52 As a reflector recedes from a transducer at 50 cm/s, the round-trip distance between them is increased at the rate _____ cm/s.

4.53 Exercises 4.51 and 4.52 present one reason why there is a factor of _____ in the doppler equation for a reflector.

4.54 Figure 4.13 shows a police radar unit (P) using the doppler effect to determine the speed of an automobile (A). What happens to the doppler shift as the vehicle travels down the highway?

Chapter 5

Doppler Instruments

Four types of instruments are used for doppler detection of flow in the heart, arteries, and veins. The continuous-wave instrument detects doppler-shifted echoes in the region of overlap between the beams of the transmitting transducer and the receiving transducer elements. In principle, it has an unlimited doppler shift frequency operating range. Transducers are discussed in Section 2.2. The primary difference between transducers designed for imaging and those designed for doppler use is that the latter are not damped (and are, therefore, more efficient). This is because they emit longer pulses than those used in imaging. The pulsed-wave doppler instrument emits ultrasound pulses and receives echoes from a single transducer element and beam. Through range gating it provides the ability to select doppler information from a particular location within the anatomy. To use the pulsed-wave doppler intelligently it is usually combined with real-time sonography in one instrument. Such instruments are called duplex scanners because of their dual functions (imaging and flow measurement). Color-flow doppler instruments provide two-dimensional, real-time, color-coded doppler information superimposed on the real-time, gray-scale anatomic display. The color coding provides information regarding flow direction and, sometimes, other characteristics. These instrument types are described in detail in the following sections.

5.1
Continuous Wave

Ultrasound doppler instruments must provide continuous or pulsed voltages to the transducer and convert voltages received from the transducer to audible or visual information corresponding to reflector or scatterer motion. If an instrument can distinguish between positive and negative doppler shifts, it is said to be bidirectional. Continuous-wave doppler instruments consist of a continuous-wave voltage generator and a receiver that detects the change in frequency (doppler shift) resulting from reflector or scatterer motion for presentation as an audible sound and an image corresponding to motion of the objects.

A diagram of the components of a continuous-wave doppler system is given in Figure 5.1. The voltage generator (oscillator) produces a continuous voltage of a frequency in the range of 2 to 10 MHz, which is applied

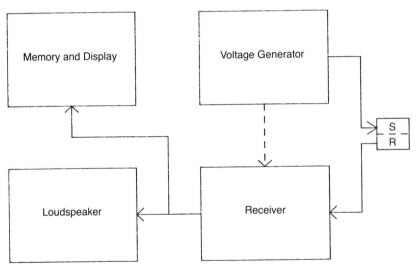

Figure 5.1. Block diagram of continuous-wave doppler instrument. The voltage generator produces a continuously alternating voltage that drives the source transducer (S). The receiving transducer (R) produces continuous voltage in response to reflections it continuously receives. The receiver detects any difference in frequency between the voltages produced by the continuous-wave generator and by the receiving transducer. The doppler shift produces a voltage that drives a loudspeaker in the audible range and a visual display. The frequency of the audible sound is equal to the doppler shift. It is proportional to the reflector speed and to the cosine of the angle between the sound propagation direction and the boundary motion.

to the source transducer. The ultrasound frequency is determined by the voltage generator. It is set to equal the operating frequency of the transducer (Section 2.2). In the transducer assembly there is a separate receiving transducer element that produces a voltage with a frequency equal to the frequency of the returning echoes. If there is reflector motion, the reflected ultrasound and the ultrasound produced by the source transducer will have different frequencies. The receiver detects the difference between these two frequencies (the doppler shift) and drives a loudspeaker at this difference frequency. The doppler shift is typically one thousandth of the source frequency, which puts it in the audible range. The doppler shifts are also commonly sent to a display for visual observation and evaluation. This is discussed in Chapter 6.

The receiver amplifies the echo voltages it receives from the receiving transducer, usually determines motion direction (positive or negative doppler shift), and acquires (demodulates) the doppler shift information in the returning echoes. Although continuous-wave receivers do not have time-gain compensation (attenuation compensation), pulsed-wave and color-flow doppler instruments do. The doppler shift is derived by mixing (multiplying) the returning voltages with the continuous-wave voltage from the voltage generator (through the dashed path in Fig. 5.1). This produces the sum and difference of the voltage generator and echo frequency. The difference is the desired doppler shift. The sum is a much higher frequency (approximately double the operating frequency) and is easily filtered out. The difference is zero for echoes returning from stationary structures. For echoes from moving structures or flowing blood, this difference is the doppler shift that provides information on motion and flow.

Determining direction (positive versus negative doppler shifts) and separating doppler shift voltages into separate forward and reverse channels is accomplished by the phase-quadrature detector. Two voltages from the voltage generator (one delayed by one quarter of a cycle, i.e., "quad") are mixed with the returning echo voltages yielding the difference (doppler shifts). These two signals are then demodulated by rectification and filtering as described in Section 2.3. One signal is then delayed by one quarter of a cycle, and the two signals are then fed to an adder and to a subtracter. The subtracter provides the forward (positive doppler shift) channel while the adder provides the reverse (negative doppler shift) channel. These two signals can then be applied to separate loudspeakers or headphones and to the positive (above baseline) and negative (below baseline) portion of a spectral display.

Simpler systems, such as the hand-held, nondirectional device, only yield an audible output. Analogue zero-crossing detector devices provide a single value (an average of some sort) for doppler shift as a function of time. This is usually fed to a strip chart recorder that produces hard copy

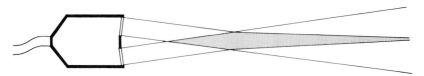

Figure 5.2. Continuous-wave doppler systems have dual-element transducer assemblies, one for transmitting and one for receiving. The region over which doppler information can be acquired (doppler sample volume) is the region of transmitting and receiving beam overlap (shaded region).

of the average doppler shift versus time. Direction is indicated above and below a zero baseline. The zero-crossing detector counts how often the signal voltage changes from negative to positive. The higher the count, the higher the frequency. This count is presented on the vertical axis of a two-dimensional graph where horizontal axis represents time.

Doppler receivers often have a reject or threshold function (Section 2.3) for elimination of weaker intensity doppler signals. Thus, the doppler receiver has essentially the same functions as the imaging receiver described in Section 2.3 with the addition of the detection of doppler shift magnitude and sign.

A continuous-wave instrument detects flow that occurs anywhere within the intersection of the transmit and receive beams of the dual-transducer assembly (Fig. 5.2). The doppler sample volume (the region from which doppler-shifted echoes return and are presented audibly or visually) is the overlapping region of the transmit and receive beams.

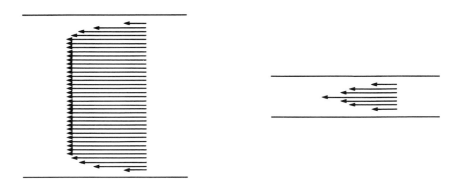

A   B

Figure 5.3. The flow profile is more uniform in *A,* a large-diameter vessel, than it is in *B,* a small one. (From Kremkau FW: Technical considerations, equipment, and physics of duplex sonography. *In* Grant EG, White EM: Duplex Sonography. New York, Springer-Verlag, 1988. Reprinted with permission.)

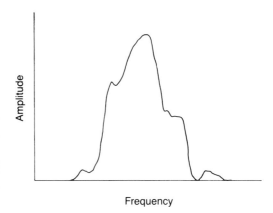

Figure 5.4. A frequency spectrum plot of the amplitude of each frequency component present in the returned pulses. Many frequencies are present because of the distribution of flow speeds encountered by the beam in the vessel.

Because the sample volume is rather large, continuous-wave doppler systems can give complicated and confusing presentations if reflectors or scatterers with different motions or flows are included in the sound beams (e.g., two blood vessels being viewed simultaneously). Pulsed-doppler systems help solve this problem by monitoring motion or flow at selected distances or depths with relatively small sample volumes.

Because a distribution of flow velocities is encountered by the sound pulses as they traverse a vessel (Fig. 5.3), a distribution of many doppler-shifted frequencies returns to the transducer and the instrument (Fig. 5.4). As a presentation like Figure 5.4 is continuously changing with cardiac cycle, it can be displayed as a function of time with appropriate real-time frequency spectrum processing (Figs. 5.5 and 5.6). These displays provide

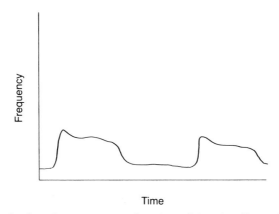

Figure 5.5. A display of spectrum as a function of time (cardiac cycle). Frequency is now on the vertical axis. The amplitude of each frequency component at each instant of time is represented by gray level or color.

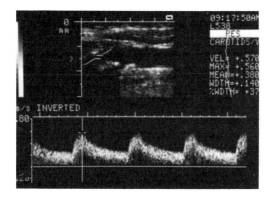

Figure 5.6. Clinical example (carotid artery) of a display of doppler spectrum as a function of time. (Courtesy of Acuson.)

quantitative data for evaluating doppler-shifted echoes otherwise presented audibly. The fast fourier transform (FFT) is the mathematical technique[41] the instrument uses to derive the doppler spectrum from the returning echoes of various frequencies. These displays can show spectral broadening, which is the widening of the doppler shift spectrum, i.e., the increase of the range of doppler shift frequencies present, due to a broader range of flow speeds and directions encountered by the sound beam. This occurs for normal flow in smaller vessels and for disturbed and turbulent flow in any vessel. Further detail on this topic is presented in Chapter 6.

To convert a spectral display correctly from doppler shift versus time to flow speed versus time, the doppler angle must be accurately incorporated into the calculation process (Section 4.3). The display is a cathode-ray tube discussed in Section 2.3. The displayed anatomic and doppler information is normally stored in a digital memory (Section 2.3) before display.

To eliminate the high-intensity, low-frequency doppler shift echoes (wall thump) resulting from heart or vessel wall motion with pulsatile flow, a high-pass wall filter (that rejects frequencies below an adjustable value) is used. Sometimes called a wall-thump filter, it rejects these strong echoes that would overwhelm the weaker echoes from the blood. The lower-limit range of the filter is about 50 to 3200 Hz. Caution should be used with the filter because it can affect pulsatility index calculations (see Fig. 6.18).

5.2
Pulsed Wave

A diagram of the components of a pulsed-doppler (pulsed-wave) instrument is given in Figure 5.7. The voltage generator is similar to that

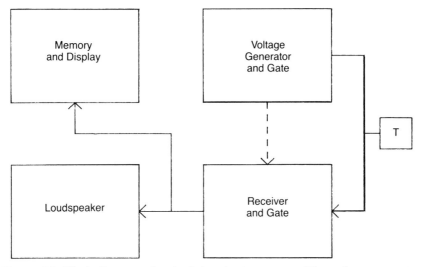

Figure 5.7. Block diagram of pulsed-doppler instrument. The voltage generator produces a continuously alternating voltage. The generator gate converts this continuous voltage to voltage pulses that drive the transducer (T). This is normally a single-element transducer. Received pulses are delivered to the receiver, where their frequencies are compared with the generator frequency. The difference (doppler shift) is sent to the loudspeaker and display. The receiver also contains a gate that selects reflections from a given depth according to arrival time and thus gives motion information as a function of depth. (From Kremkau FW: Technical considerations, equipment, and physics of duplex sonography. *In* Grant EG, White EM: Duplex Sonography. New York, Springer-Verlag, 1988. Reprinted with permission.)

in Figure 5.1. The generator gate allows pulses of a few cycles of voltage to pass on to the transducer where ultrasound pulses are produced. As discussed in Chapter 2, imaging pulses are two or three cycles long. Pulses used in pulsed doppler instruments, however, have minimum pulse lengths of about five cycles. This is necessary to determine doppler shift of returning echoes properly. Pulses may be as long as 25 or 30 cycles. The transducer assembly contains only one transducer element, which functions as both the source and receiving transducer. Voltage pulses resulting from received echoes are processed in the receiver. The frequency of the pulses is compared with the voltage generator frequency, and the doppler shift magnitude and sign derived as described in Section 5.1. The doppler shift signal is sent to loudspeakers for an audible output and to the display for visual output. Based on their arrival time, echoes coming from reflectors at a given depth may be selected by the receiver gate; thus, motion information may be obtained as a function of depth. Receiver gate length and location (depth into tissue) are controllable by the operator.

Table 5.1
Echo Arrival Time (t) for Various
Reflector Depths (d)

d (cm)	t (μs)
0.5	6.5
1.0	13.0
2.0	26.0
4.0	52.0
8.0	104.0
15.0	195.0
20.0	260.0

(From Kremkau FW: Technical considerations, equipment, and physics of duplex
sonography. *In* Grant EG, White EM:
Duplex Sonography. New York, Springer-
Verlag, 1988. Reprinted with permission.)

There is an upper limit to doppler shift that can be detected by pulsed
instruments, which is one half the pulse repetition frequency (in the range
of 5 to 30 kHz). When this limit (sometimes called the nyquist limit) is
exceeded, aliasing occurs (Section 7.1). Improper doppler shift information
(improper direction and improper value) results. An analogous optical
form of aliasing occurs in motion pictures when wagon wheels appear to
rotate at various speeds and in reverse direction. Higher pulse repetition
frequencies permit higher doppler shifts to be detected but also increase
the chance of range ambiguity artifact (Section 7.1). Continuous-wave
doppler instruments do not have this limitation (but neither do they provide any depth information).

A single receiver gate selects one listening region from which returning doppler-shifted echoes are accepted (Table 5.1 and Figs. 5.8 through

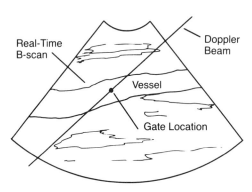

Figure 5.8. Image from a combined real-time and pulsed-
doppler instrument. The doppler
receiver gate can be located visually inside a vessel. Figure 5.6
shows such an image from the
display of a pulsed-wave instrument.

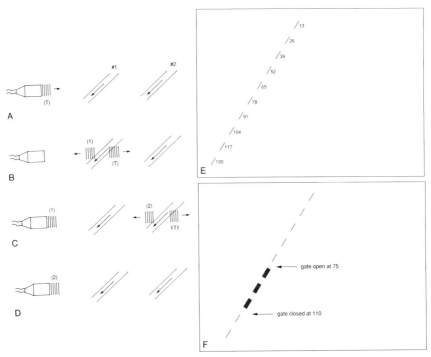

Figure 5.9. (a) A pulse (T) leaves the transducer; (b) an echo (1) is generated in vessel #1; (c) echo (1) arrives at the transducer. At the same time, another echo (2) is generated at vessel #2; (d) echo (2) arrives at the transducer after echo (1) did (c). These echoes will be processed by the instrument if the receiver gate is open when they arrive; (e) echoes from 1, 2, 3, 4, 5, 6, 7, 8, 9, and 10 cm depths arrive at the times (μs) indicated. (f) If the gate is open from 75 to 110 μs after pulse emission, only echoes arriving at 78, 91, and 104 μs will be accepted. The others in (e) will be rejected.

5.10). The gate has some length (depth range) over which it permits reception (Table 5.2). For example (using the rule: 13 μs round-trip travel time per centimeter of depth—Section 2.1), a gate that passes echoes arriving from 13 to 15 μs after pulse generation is effectively listening at a depth range of 10.0 to 11.6 mm. In this case the gate is located at a depth of 10.8 mm with a length (depth range) of ± 0.8 mm. Generally, larger gate lengths (e.g., 10 mm) are used when searching for the desired vessel and flow and then shorter gate lengths (e.g., 3 mm) for spectral analysis (Chapter 6) and evaluation. The shorter gate length improves the signal-to-noise ratio and the quality of the spectral trace. A single gate allows only one depth and length selection (from which all doppler-shifted echoes will be accepted in combination) at any time. To receive and separate doppler

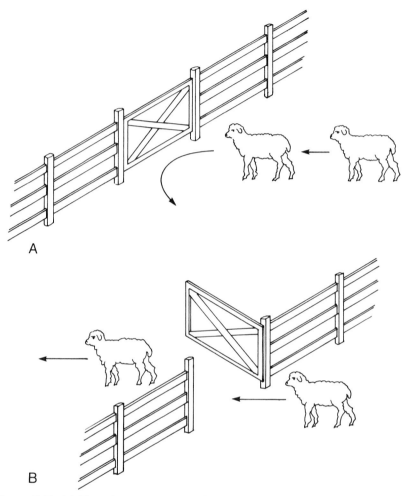

Figure 5.10. (a) Two sheep arrive at a closed gate and are not received into the pen; (b) two sheep arrive later at the gate when it is open and are received. In a doppler receiver the gate accepts and rejects echoes in a similar manner.

information simultaneously from several depths (e.g., to obtain a flow profile across a vessel), multiple gates must be used. These separate the doppler information from several depths into separate channels for processing and display.

The doppler sample volume (the region from which doppler-shifted echoes return and are presented audibly or visually) is determined by the beam width, the receiver gate length, and the emitted pulse length. One

Table 5.2
Spatial Gate Length (L) for Various
Temporal Gate Lengths (T)*

T (μs)	L (mm)
1.3	1
2.6	2
6.5	5
13.0	10

*Time from gate turn-on to turn-off. This table assumes zero pulse length. (From Kremkau FW: Technical considerations, equipment, and physics of duplex sonography. *In* Grant EG, White EM: Duplex Sonography. New York, Springer-Verlag, 1988. Reprinted with permission.)

half the pulse length is added to gate length to yield the effective sample volume length. Thus, the pulse length must shorten as gate length is reduced. The sample volume width is equal to the beam width at the sample volume depth location.

Volume flow (mL/s) can be calculated from mean speed multiplied by vessel cross-sectional area. To do this correctly, the various doppler shifts representing the cells moving at various speeds must be averaged properly, the angle properly accounted for to convert mean doppler shift to mean speed, and the area correctly determined from a vessel diameter measurement aided by the operator (Fig. 5.11) and assuming circular cross-section. Clearly, several things can go wrong in this process, yielding faulty results.[42]

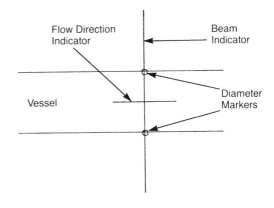

Figure 5.11. A duplex doppler instrument display usually has operator-controllable indicators for flow direction and vessel diameter. (From Kremkau FW: Technical considerations, equipment, and physics of duplex sonography. *In* Grant EG, White EM: Duplex Sonography. New York, Springer-Verlag, 1988. Reprinted with permission.)

Flow Direction Indicator

Beam Indicator

Vessel

Diameter Markers

5.3
Duplex

Combinations of instruments discussed in Sections 2.3, 5.1, and 5.2 are available commercially. Pulsed and continuous-wave doppler systems are available in the same instrument. Real-time cross-sectional ultrasound imaging instruments are available with pulsed doppler or both continuous and pulsed doppler. These provide the capability of imaging anatomic structures as well as analyzing motion and flow at a known point in the anatomic field (see Figs. 5.6 and 5.12). Doppler angle can be visually accounted for (Fig. 5.12a and b) but can also be erroneously handled (Fig. 5.12c). Imaging allows intelligent positioning of the gate in a pulsed-wave doppler system. The availability of continuous-wave and pulsed-wave doppler in the same system is useful because difficulty is encountered in a pulsed system if the flow rates become so high that the doppler shift exceeds half the pulse repetition frequency (aliasing) (Section 7.1). At that point, the ability to shift to the continuous-wave system (even though it means giving up depth information) is advantageous.

Duplex systems must be time-shared. That is, imaging and doppler flow measurements cannot be done simultaneously. Systems using mechanical transducers (see Fig. 2.25) must stop the transducer movement to perform the doppler function. The anatomic image is frozen on the display during doppler acquisition. Electronic scanning with arrays (see Figs. 2.26–2.29) permits rapid switching between imaging and doppler functions (several times per second), allowing apparent simultaneous acquisition of real-time image and doppler flow information (see Fig. 5.6). Imaging frame rates are slowed to allow for interlaced acquisition of doppler information.

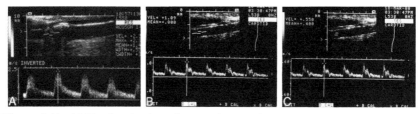

Figure 5.12. (a) Duplex display of internal-carotid artery stenosis with angle-corrected pulsed-doppler spectrum (courtesy of Acuson); (b) angle-corrected flow speed measurement (1.09 m/s) in the carotid artery; (c) uncorrected measurement erroneously indicating 0.55 m/s. (b and c from Taylor KJW, Holland S: Doppler ultrasound I. Basic principles, instrumentation and pitfalls. Radiology 174:297–307, 1990. Reprinted with permission.)

5.4
Color Flow

The continuous-wave and pulsed-wave instruments described in the previous sections are limited to a presentation of real-time, doppler-shift information from a relatively localized region within tissue (overlapping beams region or sample volume). As discussed previously, this is normally presented as a plot of doppler shift versus time. It is also possible to display doppler flow information in a manner similar to real-time, two-dimensional sonography of anatomic structures. This is accomplished using a pulse-echo technique similar to that for gray-scale imaging. That is, pulses are sent through all regions of the anatomic field from which flow information is desired. But rather than displaying returning echoes with gray-scale brightnesses corresponding to their intensities, as in anatomic imaging, echoes are displayed with colors (see Color Plates II and III) corresponding to the direction of flow that their positive or negative doppler shifts represent (toward or away from the transducer). The brightness of the color can represent the intensity of the echoes, and sometimes other colors (e.g., green) are added to indicate the extent of spectral broadening or a threshold level of doppler shift being exceeded. Color choices for these applications are not standardized, and there is some debate regarding which are best.[43-47]

Approximately 10 pulses are used to obtain one line of color-flow information. (In sonography only one pulse per scan is required; see Chapter 2). There are approximately 100 to 400 doppler samples per line on a color-flow display. Depending on depth and width of the color image, 4 to 60 frames per second are produced.

The rapid rate of echo return and presentation on the display does not permit determination of the doppler spectrum using the fourier transform technique. There is no way to present this two-dimensional information (doppler shift versus time) at every point on a two-dimensional display, anyway. Instead, other techniques are used. Autocorrelation is the common one in which each echo is correlated with the corresponding one from the previous pulse, thus determining the motion that has occurred during each pulse period. At least three pulses are required to do this. A real-time value for mean flow speed is produced. As this is positive or negative with respect to flow direction, it is possible to present real-time, color-coded flow direction information two-dimensionally on the display. This is normally superimposed on the two-dimensional, gray-scale anatomic scan. Examples are given in Color Plates IV and V. The aliasing artifact appears in these displays as a region of different color (opposite flow) where the doppler shift exceeds half the pulse repetition frequency (see

Color Plate V). Color Plate VIa shows an example of lack of flow (color) due to a 90-degree doppler angle. With an acceptable angle (Color Plate VIb), flow is detected. Color Plate VII shows examples of flow reversal in the normal carotid bulb and color flow with doppler spectrum in the brachial artery. Color Plate VIII shows color-flow examples in an aortic aneurysm and inferior vena cava and in the iliac bifurcation. Color Plate IX shows cardiac color-flow examples with the effect of wall-filter setting. Color Plate X shows eddy currents due to atheroma.

5.5
Review

Doppler instruments make use of the doppler shift to yield information regarding motion and flow. Continuous-wave systems provide motion and flow information without depth information or selection capability. Pulsed-doppler systems provide depth information and the ability to select depth from which doppler information is received. Spectral analysis provides visual information on the distribution of received doppler-shift frequencies resulting from the distribution of scatterer velocities (speeds and directions) encountered. In addition to audible output, imaging of vessel flow spectra is possible in doppler systems. Combined systems utilizing dynamic sonography and continuous-wave and pulsed-wave doppler are available commercially. Color-flow systems provide displays of two-dimensional, real-time flow superimposed on gray-scale anatomic scans. Flow direction is indicated by the color assignment to the doppler-shifted echoes on the display.

Exercises

5.1 All doppler instruments distinguish between positive and negative doppler shifts. True or false?

5.2 Instruments that distinguish between positive and negative doppler shifts yield motion _____ information and are called _____.

5.3 Continuous-wave doppler instruments use single-element transducers similar to those used in imaging. True or false?

5.4 The components of a continuous-wave doppler system include

_____ _____, _____

_____, _____, _____,

_____, _____,

and _____.

5.5 Quantitative information about the frequencies contained in returning doppler-shifted echoes can be displayed on an _____ versus _____ plot that is continuously changing with time.

5.6 To display the pattern of time change of a doppler spectrum, a display of _____ versus _____ can be used.

5.7 In Exercise 5.6 the amplitude of each frequency component is represented by _____ level or _____.

5.8 The received frequency spectrum exists (rather than a single frequency) because of the distribution of _____ _____ encountered by the ultrasound.

5.9 Because velocity is speed and direction, variations in either of these in the flow region monitored by the doppler instrument may contribute to the received frequency spectrum. True or false?

5.10 The components of a pulsed-doppler instrument are the same as those for a continuous-wave instrument except for the addition of two _____ and the combining of two _____ into one.

5.11 The purpose of the generator gate is to convert a _____ voltage to a _____ voltage.

5.12 The purpose of the receiver gate is to allow selection of doppler-shifted echoes from specific _____ according to _____ _____.

5.13 Pulsed-doppler instruments require a two-element transducer assembly. True or false?

5.14 Multiple gates provide motion or flow _____ information.

5.15 A later receiver gate corresponds to a deeper gate location. True or false?

5.16 There is no problem with aliasing as long as the doppler shifts are _____ half the pulse repetition frequency.
   a. less than
   b. equal to
   c. greater than
   d. all of the above
   e. a or b

5.17 To receive and display doppler information simultaneously from several depths, several _____ must be used in the receiver.

5.18 Color-flow instruments present two-dimensional, color-coded images representing _____ that are superimposed on gray-scale images representing _____.

5.19 Which of the following on a color-flow display is (are) presented in real-time?
  a. gray-scale anatomy
  b. flow direction
  c. doppler spectrum
  d. a and b
  e. all of the above

5.20 If red represents flow toward the transducer and blue represents flow away, what color would be seen for normal flow toward the transducer? What color would be seen for aliasing flow toward the transducer? What colors for normal flow away and for aliasing flow away?

5.21 Pulsed-doppler instruments use the _____ _____ _____ technique to yield doppler shift spectra as a function of time.

5.22 Color-flow instruments use an _____ technique to yield _____ flow speed in real-time.

5.23 The fourier transform technique is not used in color-flow instruments because it is not _____ enough.
  a. slow
  b. fast
  c. bright
  d. cheap
  e. none of the above

5.24 The abbreviation for the technique referred to in Exercise 5.21 is _____.

5.25 Do the different colors appearing in Color Plate VIII indicate that flow is going in two different directions in each vessel?

5.26 In Figure 5.6 is the instrument a pulsed-wave or continuous-wave device?

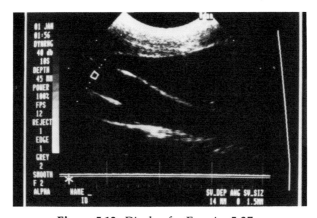

Figure 5.13. Display for Exercise 5.27.

5.27 In Figure 5.13 is the instrument used a pulsed-wave or continuous-wave device?

5.28 If a sheep leaves its pen and runs to another pen 25 meters distant at a speed of 50 cm/s, when must the gate to the second pen open to allow the sheep to pass through when it arrives?

5.29 If a sheep leaves its pen and travels to a brook at which point it turns around and returns to the pen, when must the gate to its pen open to allow the sheep to pass through when it returns? (Distance to the brook is 25 meters, and the sheep travels at 50 cm/s.)

5.30 Transducers designed for doppler use are generally not _____. This is because they emit _____ pulses than those used in imaging. Undamped transducers are more _____ than damped ones.

5.31 For a 5-MHz instrument and 60-degree doppler angle, a 100-Hz filter eliminates flow speeds below
   a. 1 cm/s
   b. 2 cm/s
   c. 3 cm/s
   d. 4 cm/s
   e. 5 cm/s

5.32 For a 2.5-MHz instrument and 0-degree doppler angle, a 100-Hz filter eliminates flow speeds below
   a. 1 cm/s
   b. 2 cm/s
   c. 3 cm/s
   d. 4 cm/s
   e. 5 cm/s

5.33 The functions of a doppler receiver include which of the following?
   a. amplification
   b. phase-quadrature detection
   c. demodulation
   d. rejection
   e. all of the above

5.34 An earlier receiver gate time means a _____ sample volume depth.
   a. later
   b. shallower
   c. deeper
   d. stronger
   e. none of the above

5.35 Name the four types of instruments used for doppler detection of flow.

5.36 Name the doppler instrument whose sample volume is the region of transmitting and receiving transducer beam overlap.

5.37 Name the instrument whose sample volume is determined by the receiver gate.

5.38 Name the instrument that combines pulsed-doppler with imaging.

5.39 Name the instrument that presents two-dimensional doppler information superimposed on an anatomic image.

5.40 The _____ detects the difference between the frequencies of the emitted and received ultrasound.

5.41 The doppler shift is typically _____ of the source frequency.
  a. $\frac{1}{1000}$th
  b. $\frac{1}{100}$th
  c. $\frac{1}{10}$th
  d. 10 times
  e. 100 times

5.42 To convert a spectral display correctly from doppler shift to flow speed, the _____ _____ must be accurately incorporated.

5.43 The doppler spectrum is visually presented on a _____-_____ tube.

5.44 The high-pass filter in the receiver is called a _____ filter or _____-_____ filter.

5.45 Pulsed-doppler instruments produce pulses that are about _____ to _____ cycles long. The length of the sample volume in a pulsed-doppler instrument is determined by the receiver _____ length and the emitted _____ length.

5.46 The doppler shift upper limit to avoid aliasing is sometimes called the _____ limit.

5.47 If aliasing is avoided by increasing pulse repetition frequency, name the other artifact that may be encountered.

5.48 Which type of doppler instrument is most likely to be used in measuring extremely high flow rates?

5.49 All pulsed instruments have anatomic imaging capability to allow intelligent positioning of the gate. True or false?

5.50 Continuous-wave and pulsed-wave doppler capabilities are never provided in the same instrument. True or false?

5.51 Which type of duplex system cannot image while doppler information is being acquired?

5.52 In color-flow instruments color is used only to represent flow direction. True or false?

5.53 Two or three cycle-long pulses are used for
  a. pulsed-doppler
  b. continuous-wave doppler

    c. imaging

    d. color-flow doppler

    e. all of the above

5.54 Approximately _____ pulses are required to obtain one line of color-flow information.

    a. 1

    b. 10

    c. 100

    d. 1000

    e. 1,000,000

5.55 There are approximately _____ samples per line on a color-flow display.

    a. 2

    b. 20

    c. 200

    d. 2000

    e. 2,000,000

5.56 There are about _____ frames per second produced by a color-flow doppler instrument.

    a. 10

    b. 20

    c. 40

    d. 80

    e. more than one of the above

5.57 Which of the following instruments can produce aliasing?

    a. continuous-wave doppler

    b. pulsed-doppler

    c. duplex

    d. color-flow

    e. more than one of the above

5.58 Color-flow displays are not dependent on the doppler angle. True or false?

5.59 If two colors are shown in the same vessel using a color-flow instrument, it always means flow is occurring in opposite directions in the vessel. True or false?

Chapter 6

Spectral Analysis

Spectral means relating to a spectrum. A spectrum is an array of the components of a wave separated and arranged in order of increasing wavelength or frequency. Analysis comes from a Greek word meaning to break up. Thus, spectral analysis is the breaking up of the components of a complex wave or signal and spreading out the components in order.

A prism does this for light. When white light passes through a prism, it is separated into a sequence of the various colors making up the white appearance. White light is a combination of the full range of frequencies visible to the human eye. Frequency is interpreted as color by the brain with red being the lowest frequency and violet being the highest. The prism breaks up these frequency components and spreads them out so that the various colors are seen in what is called a color spectrum. A similar process is performed electronically for the returning echoes in a doppler system. This is introduced in Section 5.1.

The human auditory system does this for sound. The ear and brain break down the complex sounds we receive into the component frequencies present. Thus, we can listen to a doppler signal and recognize normal and abnormal sounds. Visual presentation of these sounds provides additional capability for recognition of flow characteristics and diagnosis of disease. The visual presentation and interpretation of doppler spectral information is considered in detail in this chapter.

6.1
Spectrum Source

In Chapter 3, flow profiles in vessels were described. It was seen that the character of the flow profiles was determined by the size of the vessel and the uniformity of its wall. Changes in size, turns, and abnormalities, such as presence of plaque and stenoses, alter the flow character. We have seen that flow can be characterized as plug, laminar, disturbed, and turbulent. In all cases (even for normal steady flow), portions of the flowing fluid within a vessel are moving at different speeds and, sometimes, in different directions. Thus, as the ultrasound beam intersects this flow and echoes are produced, many different doppler shifts are received from the vessel by the system. If all the blood cells were flowing at the same speed, a single doppler shift would result. However, this is not the case. The extent of the range of generated doppler shift frequencies depends upon the character of the flow. For near-plug flow (normal flow in a large vessel, particularly in systole), a narrow range of doppler-shift frequencies is received. In diastole, in smaller vessels, and in disturbed and turbulent flow, much broader ranges of doppler-shift frequencies can be received. Other vessels can have an intermediate flow character called blunted parabolic flow.

6.2
Spectral Trace

The received doppler signal is a combination of many doppler shift frequencies yielding a complicated waveform (Fig. 6.1a). Using the fast fourier transform (Section 5.1), these frequencies are separated into a spectrum that can be presented on a two-dimensional display as doppler-shift frequency on the horizontal axis and power or amplitude of each frequency component on the vertical axis (Figs. 6.1b and 6.2). For venous flow such a spectrum would commonly be rather constant. However, for the pulsatile flow in arterial circulation, such a presentation would be continually changing—shifting to the right in systole as the blood accelerates and doppler shifts increase, shifting to the left in diastole, and changing in power or amplitude over the cardiac cycle. The interpretation of this

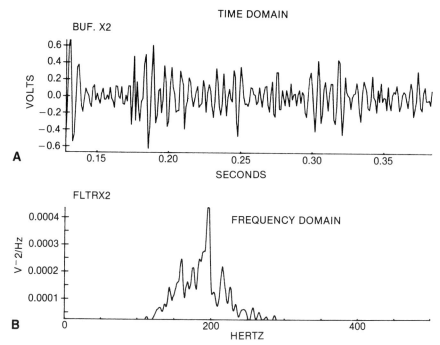

Figure 6.1. (a) Demodulated doppler shift signal for microspheres flowing at nearly uniform speed. When applied to a loudspeaker, a mix of many frequencies is heard. Approximately 10 cycles occur over the time period 0.20 to 0.25 seconds. Thus, the fundamental period of this signal is about 50 ms yielding a fundamental frequency of 200 Hz. (b) After the fourier transform is applied, a frequency spectrum is obtained. The center frequency is approximately 200 Hz. This is what was predicted in part (a). (From Burns PN: The physical principles of doppler and spectral analysis. J Clin Ultrasound 15:567–590, 1987. Reprinted with permission.)

changing presentation is difficult and, indeed, the character of the changes over cardiac cycle could be important. Therefore, presentation of this changing spectrum as a function of time is valuable and useful. Such a trace is shown in Figures 6.2 and 6.3. The two display dimensions are used in this presentation as follows: The vertical axis represents doppler shift frequency, and the horizontal represents time. The amplitude or power of each doppler shift frequency component at any instant (vertical axis in Fig. 6.1b) is now presented in brightness or gray scale. Doppler signal power is proportional to blood cell density (number of cells per unit volume). A bright spot on a spectral display means that a strong doppler shift frequency component at that instant of time was received (Figs. 6.2 and 6.4). A dark spot means that a doppler shift frequency component at that point in time was weak or nonexistent. If the gray scale is reversed as in Figure

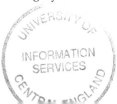

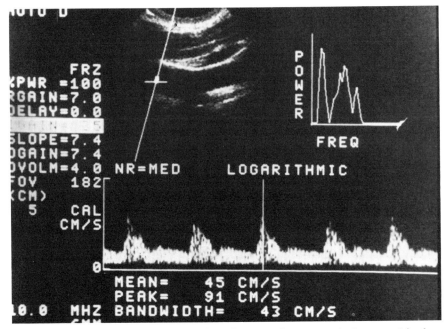

Figure 6.2. A duplex doppler display showing the anatomic image with the doppler beam line and sample gate dots (top center), doppler spectrum (top right), and spectral display (doppler shift versus time) (bottom).

6.3, bright represents weak and dark represents strong. Intermediate values of gray shade or brightness indicate intermediate amplitudes or powers of frequency components at the given times. A strong signal at a particular frequency and time means that there are many scattering blood cells moving at velocities (speeds and directions) corresponding to that doppler shift. A weak frequency (usually presented as dark) means that few cells are traveling at velocities corresponding to that doppler shift at that point in time.

6.3
Interpretation

Spectral trace presentations provide information about flow that can be used to discern conditions at the site of measurement and distal to it[48-53] (Color Plate XI). The evaluation of stenosis in the carotid artery is an example of the former. Observations of the peak flow speeds and spectral

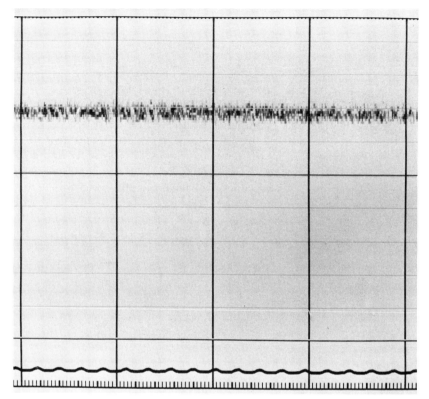

Figure 6.3. A spectral display of the signal shown in Figure 6.1. The flow is constant yielding doppler shift frequencies around 200 Hz (horizontal markers represent 100 Hz). (From Burns PN: The physical principles of doppler and spectral analysis. J Clin Ultrasound 15:567–590, 1987. Reprinted with permission.)

Figure 6.4. Four points on a spectral display: (A) and (C) occur at earlier time; (B) and (D) occur at later time; (A) and (B) are higher doppler shift frequencies while (C) and (D) are lower.

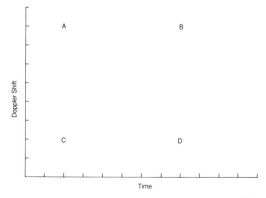

broadening are indicative of the degree of stenosis (Table 6.1). Flow speeds greater than about 120 cm/s are considered by some to be hemodynamically significant. Spectral broadening means a vertical thickening of the spectral trace (Figs. 6.5 and 6.6). If all the cells were moving at the same speed, a single doppler shift frequency would be received and the spectral trace would be a thin line (see Fig. 5.5). As described in Section 6.2, this is not found in practice. However, narrow spectra can be observed, particularly in large vessels in systole (see Figs. 3.10 and 6.7a). The apparent narrowing of the spectrum as the blood accelerates in systole can be misinterpreted. A spectrum of consistent width appears to be thinner in a steep rise portion of a curve (Fig. 6.8). As flow is disturbed or becomes turbulent, greater variation in velocities of various portions of the flowing blood produce a greater range of doppler shift frequencies. This results in a broader spectrum presented on the spectral display (see Figs. 6.5 and 6.6a–d). Thus, spectral broadening is indicative of disturbed or turbulent flow and can be related to pathology (see Table 6.1). However, spectral broadening can be artificially produced by excessive doppler receiver gain (Fig. 6.6e and f).

Another term related to spectral broadening is "window." This refers to the dark (or light for white background displays) anechoic area in the lower portion of the spectral trace, particularly in systole for normal flow (Figs. 6.5a, 6.6a, and 6.7a). As flow is disturbed or becomes turbulent, spectral broadening occurs and the window is diminished or eliminated (Figs. 6.5 and 6.6). Therefore, spectral broadening and window reduction or loss are equivalent terms.

Table 6.1
5-MHz Doppler Criteria for Carotid Stenosis*

Diameter Reduction (Percent)	Peak Systolic Flow Speed (cm/s)	Peak Diastolic Flow Speed (cm/s)	Spectral Broadening (cm/s)
0	<125	<40	<30
25	<125	<40	<40
50	>125	40	<40
75	>125	>40	>40
90	>135	>100	>80
100	0	0	0

*Modified from Roederer GO, Langlois YE, Chan AW, et al: Ultrasonic duplex scanning of extracranial carotid arteries: Improved accuracy using new features from the common carotid artery. J Cardiovasc Ultrasonography 1:373–380, 1982; Roederer GO, Langlois YE, Jager KA, et al: A simple spectral parameter for accurate classification of severe carotid disease. Bruit 8:174–178, 1984; Bluth EI, Stavros AT, Marich KW, et al: Carotid duplex sonography: a multicenter recommendation for standardized imaging and doppler criteria. RadioGraphics 8:487–506, 1988.

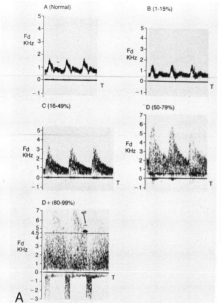
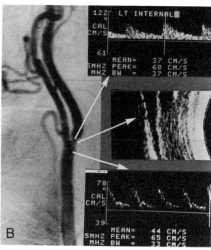

Figure 6.5. (a) Spectral displays for various degrees of carotid stenosis. (From Taylor DC, Strandness DE: Carotid artery duplex scanning. J Clin Ultrasound 15:635–644, 1987. Reprinted with permission.) (b) Montage of angiogram with slight stenosis at the origin of the internal carotid. The common carotid waveform is normal. A small plaque on the vessel wall giving rise to turbulence is seen on the ultrasound image. This results in "spectral broadening," which causes filling in of the normal clear "window" under the time-velocity waveform. Turbulence results in red cells moving at all different velocities and hence causes the spectral spread. (From Taylor KJW, Holland S: Doppler ultrasound I. Basic Principles, instrumentation; and pitfalls. Radiology 174:297–307, 1990. Reprinted with permission.)

Narrow spectra are expected in large vessels, broad spectra in small vessels, and intermediate spectra in medium size vessels. This is shown in Figure 6.7. Using pulsed doppler to monitor flow at various sites inside a vessel, a narrow spectrum would be expected near the center of the vessel (where the cells are moving the fastest) and a broader spectrum would be expected near the walls where viscous drag is slowing the flow. This is evidenced in Figure 6.9. Complicated flow (for example, in the vicinity of the carotid bulb and flow divider) is not as easily predicted but is quite different at various sites (Fig. 6.10). Turbulent flow may occur during short portions of the cardiac cycle as high enough flow speeds are achieved. This is indicated by occasional reverse flow in Figure 6.11. Spectral broadening does not necessarily indicate turbulence. Figure 6.12 shows a broad spectrum that is probably not due to disturbed or turbulent flow but simply

Text continued on page 133

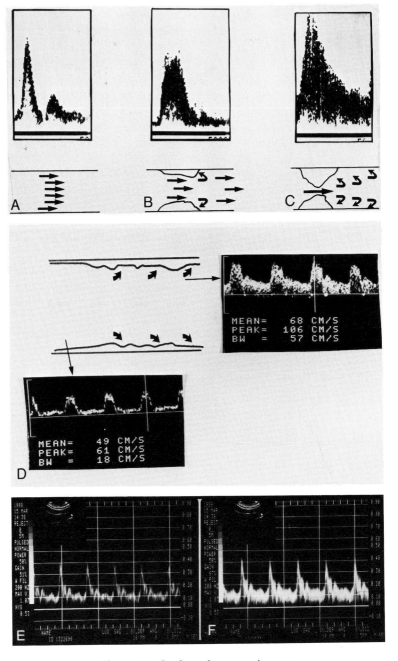

Figure 6.6 *See legend on opposite page*

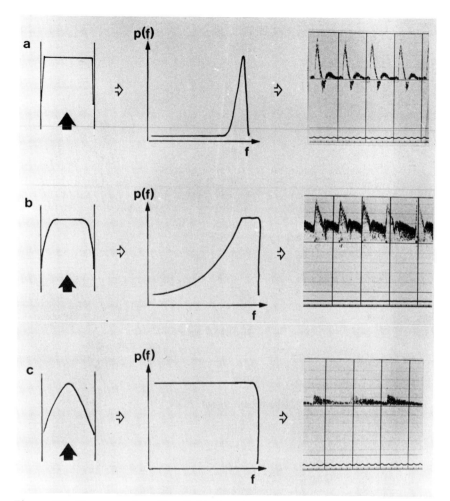

Figure 6.7. Flow speed profiles (left), doppler spectra (power versus frequency) (center), and spectral displays (right) for (a) plug flow in the aorta, (b) blunted parabolic flow in the celiac trunk, and (c) parabolic flow in the ovarian artery. (From Burns PN: The physical principles of doppler and spectral analysis. J Clin Ultrasond 15:567–590, 1987. Reprinted with permission.)

Figure 6.6. (a) With normal flow and plug or blunt flow speed profile there is a window during systole. (b) Disturbed flow produces spectral broadening. (c) Significant stenosis produces much spectral broadening and altered waveform shape. (a–c from Burns PN: The physical principles of doppler and spectral analysis. J Clin Ultrasound 15:567–590, 1987. Reprinted with permission.) (d) Spectral broadening produced by atheroma. (e) Correct doppler receiver gain setting. (f) Apparent spectral broadening caused by excessive gain. (d–f reprinted with permission. Taylor KJW, Holland S: State-of-the-art doppler ultrasound I. Basic principles, instrumentation and pitfalls. Radiology 174:297–307, 1990.)

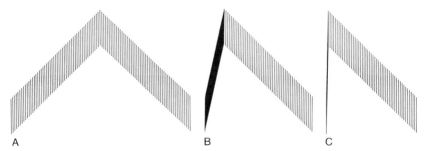

A   B   C

Figure 6.8. Apparent spectral narrowing in rapidly accelerating flow. (a) Slowly accelerating and decelerating flow shows that the spectral widths (bandwidths) are all equal. In (b) and (c), as the acceleration phase becomes steeper it appears to have a narrower bandwidth. However, the vertical lines representing bandwidth in all cases are the same.

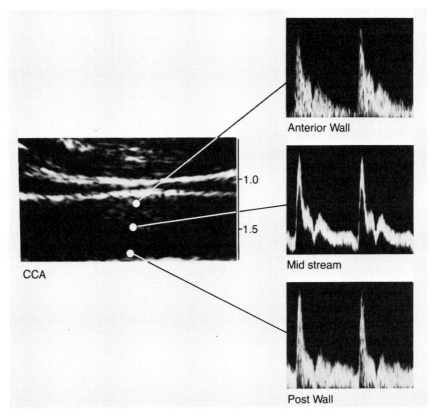

Figure 6.9. Spectral traces showing increased spectral bandwidth near vessel walls in the common carotid artery. As expected, a narrower bandwidth is found at midstream. (From Taylor DC, Strandness DE: Carotid artery duplex scanning. J Clin Ultrasound 15:635–644, 1987. Reprinted with permission.)

130

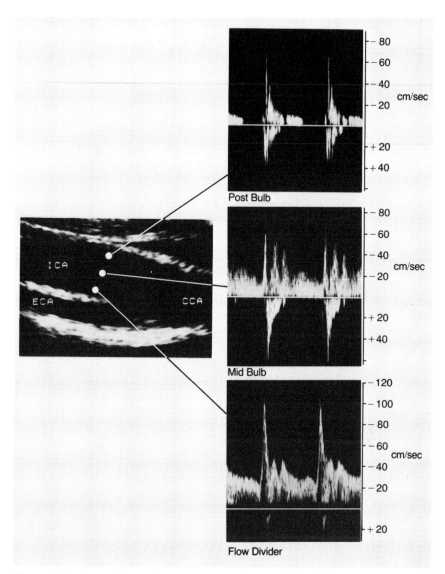

Figure 6.10. Spectral waveforms show laminar flow with mild spectral broadening adjacent to the carotid bifurcation and areas of increasing turbulence and boundary layer separation along the outer aspect of the carotid bulb. (From Taylor DC, Strandness DE: Carotid artery duplex scanning. J Clin Ultrasound 15:635–644, 1987. Reprinted with permission.)

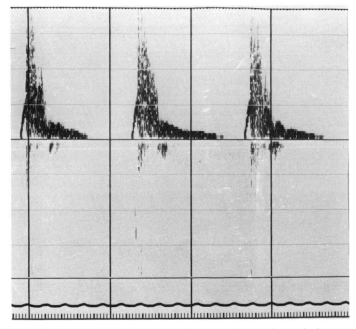

Figure 6.11. Periodic turbulence in a renal artery. During the turbulent period the peak doppler shifts are high with much spectral broadening and occasional reverse flow. (From Burns PN: The physical principles of doppler and spectral analysis. J Clin Ultrasound 15:567–590, 1987. Reprinted with permission.)

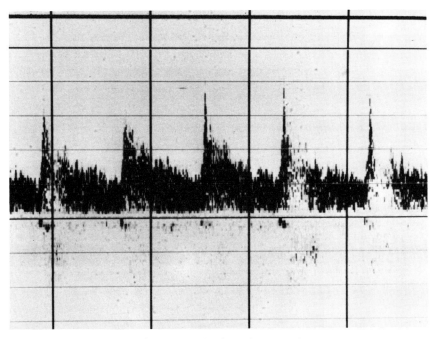

Figure 6.12 *See legend on opposite page*

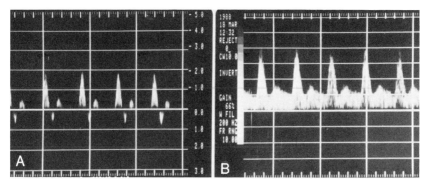

Figure 6.13. (a) High impedance flow in popliteal artery with leg at rest. (b) Low impedance flow after minimal exercise. (From Taylor KJW, Holland S: Doppler ultrasound I. Basic principles, instrumentation and pitfalls. Radiology 174:297–307, 1990. Reprinted with permission.)

due to complicated geometry, i.e., a tortuous vessel causing a variety of doppler angles and therefore a broad range (spectrum) of doppler shift frequencies.

As mentioned at the beginning of this section, doppler flow measurements can yield information regarding downstream (distal) conditions. Flow reversal in early diastole and lack of flow in late diastole (see Figs. 3.10 and 6.7a) indicate high resistance to flow downstream (e.g., due to vasoconstriction of arterioles).[24] If flow resistance is reduced because of vasodilation, impressive differences in the spectral trace are observed (Fig. 6.13). The carotid bifurcation provides an excellent site for observing expected flow characters based on normal downstream conditions. The internal carotid artery feeds a low impedance distal vascular bed (in the brain) and thus has significant diastolic flow. The external carotid artery feeds the facial vascular bed with its high impedance and thus has low diastolic flow. The common carotid artery is thus expected to have a flow characteristic of the combination of the external and internal. The three expected flow characters are seen in Figure 6.14.

Normal vessels can be occluded in diastole when pressure drops below the critical value for flow.[24] When this happens, no diastolic doppler shift will be detected. Various quantitative indices have been

Figure 6.12. Spectral trace from the splenic artery showing spectral broadening probably due to the tortuous character of the vessel. (From Burns PN: The physical principles of doppler and spectral analysis. J Clin Ultrasound 15:567–590, 1987. Reprinted with permission.)

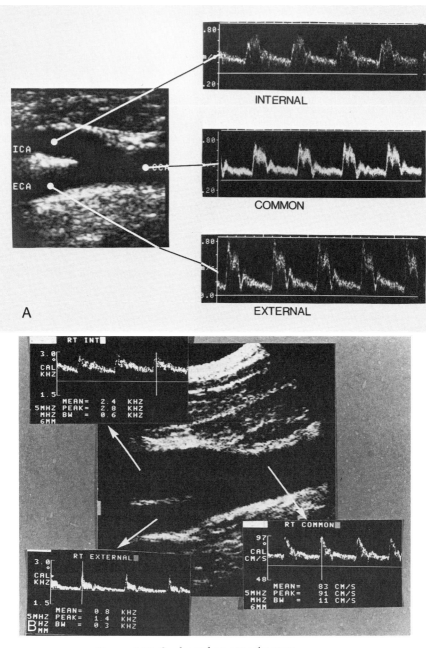

Figure 6.14 *See legend on opposite page*

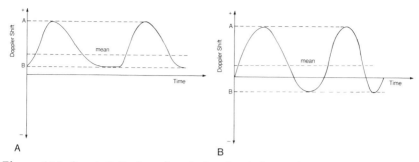

Figure 6.15. Spectral display of peak doppler shift as a function of time. A represents the maximum value at systole, and B represents the minimum value at end diastole. (a) Unidirectional flow; (b) reverse flow in diastole.

developed to describe such differences in spectral traces indicative of downstream conditions (Fig. 6.15 and Table 6.2). The differences in spectral trace shapes for high and low impedance flow and for high and low angle measurements are shown in Figure 6.16. Changing angle does not change the relationship between peak systolic and end diastolic flows. Changing distal impedance does (see Figs. 6.13 and 6.16). The pulsatility index approach works because flow impedance is not constant over cardiac cycle with distensible vessels and pulsatile pressures. That is, impedance is not constant but is greater at lower pressures and smaller at higher pressures. For rigid pipes impedance does not depend on pressure

---

Figure 6.14. (a) Common, internal, and external carotid artery spectral displays show different waveforms in accordance with downstream impedance. The low impedance flow for the internal carotid artery causes greater diastolic flow. The common carotid artery waveform is similar to the internal carotid reflecting that most of its flow goes to the internal carotid and the brain. (From Taylor DC, Strandness DE: Carotid artery duplex scanning. J Clin Ultrasound 15:635–644, 1987. Reprinted with permission.) (b) Montage to show bifurcation with corresponding doppler waveforms. The waveforms are time-velocity spectra with velocity of blood on the vertical axis and time on the horizontal axis. The clear "window" under the waveform indicates that all cells are moving at nearly the same velocity. A marker on the peak velocity indicates that the maximum velocity with the common carotid during systole is 91 cm/s. Note that there is moderate diastolic flow. The right internal carotid waveform also demonstrates a normal clear window under the time-velocity spectrum, and there is high diastolic flow. This indicates a low impedance cerebral circulation. In contrast, the waveform in the right external carotid demonstrates low diastolic flow indicating a high impedance. This difference in waveform helps to differentiate these two vessels when doubt exists. (From Taylor KJW, Burns PN, Wells PNT (eds): Clinical Applications of Doppler Ultrasound. New York, Raven Press, 1988. Reprinted with permission.)

Table 6.2
Spectral Display Indices

Name	Abbreviation	Expression*
Pulsatility Index	PI	$\dfrac{A-B}{mean}$
Resistance Index	RI	$\dfrac{A-B}{A}$
Systolic to Diastolic Ratio	SDR	$\dfrac{A}{B}$
B/A Ratio	BAR	$\dfrac{B}{A}$

*See Figure 6.15 for meaning of A and B.

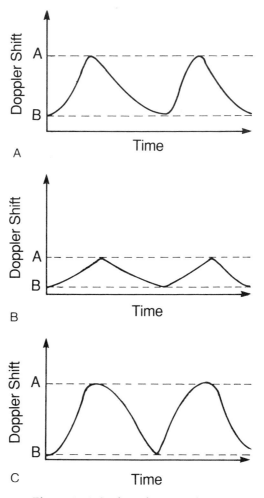

Figure 6.16 *See legend on opposite page*

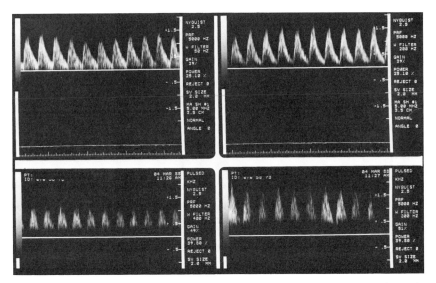

Figure 6.17. Effect of increasing the wall filter from 50 to 800 Hz simulates the appearance of a high impedance signal and will lead to misdiagnosis (e.g., of renal allograft rejection). (From Taylor KJW, Holland S: State-of-the-art doppler ultrasound I. Basic principles, instrumentation and pitfalls. Radiology 174:297–307, 1990. Reprinted with permission; courtesy of K. J. W. Taylor.)

(Poiseuille's law—Section 3.2). Care must be exercised in the use of the wall filter because it can affect the pulsatility index (Fig. 6.17).

It is important to understand that interpretation of spectral trace information can be easily oversimplified. The correlation of high flow speed with high doppler shift as shown in Figure 6.18 seems straightforward. However, this is only true if all portions of the fluid are moving parallel so that they all have the same doppler angle with the ultrasound beam. If flow is disturbed or turbulent (see Figs. 6.5 and 6.6) or if the vessel is tortuous (Fig. 6.12) or if flow is helical as claimed for the carotid,[38,39] this assumption is not valid. Then the simple interpretation is incorrect. The peak doppler shifts don't necessarily represent the fastest flow but, possibly, slow flow that is moving directly toward the transducer (small doppler angle, high doppler shift). The lowest doppler shifts do not nec-

---

Figure 6.16. (a) Spectral trace for low-impedance, low-angle flow. (b) Spectral trace for low-impedance, high-angle flow. All portions of the doppler shift are proportionally reduced. (c) Spectral trace for high-impedance, low-angle flow. Diastolic portions of the flow are reduced more than the systolic portions. This would yield a larger pulsatility index indicating higher distal flow impedance.

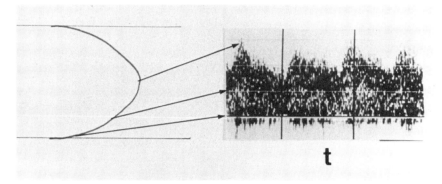

Figure 6.18. Broad spectrum of parabolic flow in a small vessel. The arrows suggest that the highest doppler shifts correspond to the fastest flow and the lowest to the slowest. This simplified approach is true only for undisturbed and nonturbulent flow where all portions of fluid are flowing parallel to each other (common doppler angle). (From Taylor KJW, Holland S: Doppler ultrasound I. Basic principles, instrumentation; and pitfalls. Radiology 174:297–307, 1990. Reprinted with permission.)

essarily represent the slowest flow but, possibly, fast flow that is moving nearly perpendicular to the beam (large doppler angle, low doppler shift). Indeed, spectral traces that have their vertical axes calibrated in speed units (usually cm/s) are only correct (Section 4.3) presentations if the doppler angle correction is proper *and* laminar undisturbed flow is being measured.

6.4
Color Flow

Because color-flow instruments use the two dimensions of their display to show two-dimensional doppler information (a flow cross section), they are unable to show spectral information in detail as described in previous sections of this chapter. Also, the autocorrelation technique (Section 5.4) does not yield the spectral detail that the fast fourier transform (Section 5.1) does. However, some measure of spectral width (for example, variance or standard deviation) can be obtained. A color tag (green, for example) can be used to indicate on the color-flow display a region where some value of this spectral index is exceeded. This tagging would indicate a region in which spectral broadening (and possibly disturbed flow or turbulence) is present.

As with the spectral trace discussed in Section 6.3, it is important not to misinterpret (oversimplify) the doppler information presented two-dimensionally in color-flow instruments. A region of bright color indicating high doppler shift is not necessarily a region of high flow speed. It could be a region of lower speed flow that is directed parallel to the beam (small doppler angle). Likewise, a dark color could indicate a region of high flow speed whose direction is nearly perpendicular to the beam. Thus, in color flow, bright does not necessarily mean fast and dark does not necessarily mean slow. Only if flow is laminar and undisturbed are these simplistic interpretations correct. Color Plate X shows a color-flow example of turbulent flow caused by atheroma.

6.5
Review

The doppler spectrum is generated by the range of scatterer velocities encountered by the ultrasound beam. It is derived electronically using the fast fourier transform and presented on the display in two forms: power versus doppler shift or doppler shift versus time with brightness indicating power. The latter presentation is, by far, the most commonly used. Flow conditions at the site of measurement are indicated by the width of the spectrum with spectral broadening and loss of window indicative of disturbed and turbulent flow. Flow conditions downstream, particularly distal flow impedance, are indicated by the relationship between peak systolic and end diastolic flow speeds. Various indices for quantitatively presenting this information have been developed. Color-flow instruments do not present spectral information in detail but can indicate regions of spectral broadening with a color tag. Oversimplistic interpretation of spectral traces and color-flow images should be avoided.

Exercises

6.1 Spectral analysis is the breaking up of the _____ of a complex wave or signal and spreading them out in _____.

6.2 Which of the following is a spectrum analyzer for light?
 a. mirror
 b. filter
 c. prism
 d. window
 e. reflector

6.3 Spectral analysis is performed in a doppler instrument
_____.
   a. electronically
   b. visually
   c. acoustically
   d. mechanically
   e. none of the above

6.4 A doppler spectrum is produced because many different doppler _____ are received from the vessel.

6.5 The statement in Exercise 6.4 is true because portions of the flowing fluid within a vessel are moving at different _____ and, sometimes, in different _____.

6.6 If all the blood cells in a vessel were moving in the same direction at the same speed, a _____ doppler shift would result.

6.7 For normal flow in a large vessel, particularly in systole, a _____ range of doppler shift frequencies is received.
   a. narrow
   b. broad
   c. steady
   d. disturbed
   e. all of the above

6.8 The type of flow in Exercise 6.7 is called _____ flow.
   a. turbulent
   b. disturbed
   c. laminar
   d. steady
   e. plug

6.9 The doppler spectrum can be presented in two ways, as a display of _____ or _____ versus doppler shift frequency or doppler shift frequency versus _____.

6.10 For pulsatile flow, in Exercise 6.9 which form of presentation is preferable, first or second?

6.11 Doppler shift versus time presentations indicate the amplitude or power of each frequency component by _____ or _____.

6.12 Doppler signal power is proportional to
   a. volume flow
   b. flow speed
   c. doppler angle
   d. cell density
   e. more than one of the above

6.13 In Figure 6.4, (A) represents
  a. early time, high doppler shift
  b. early time, low doppler shift
  c. late time, high doppler shift
  d. late time, low doppler shift
  e. none of the above

6.14 In Figure 6.4, (B) represents
  a. early time, high doppler shift
  b. early time, low doppler shift
  c. late time, high doppler shift
  d. late time, low doppler shift
  e. none of the above

6.15 In Figure 6.4, (C) represents
  a. early time, high doppler shift
  b. early time, low doppler shift
  c. late time, high doppler shift
  d. late time, low doppler shift
  e. none of the above

6.16 In Figure 6.4, (D) represents
  a. early time, high doppler shift
  b. early time, low doppler shift
  c. late time, high doppler shift
  d. late time, low doppler shift
  e. none of the above

6.17 In Figure 6.4 with a dark background, if (A) is bright, many cells are moving in such a way that a large doppler shift occurs at early time. True or false?

6.18 In Figure 6.4 with a dark background, if (D) is dark many cells are moving in such a way that they produce low doppler shifts at late time. True or false?

6.19 In the previous six exercises, high doppler shift means high flow speed only if _____ flow is assumed.

6.20 For disturbed or turbulent flow in Figure 6.4, (A) could represent
  a. high speed and large doppler angle
  b. high speed and small doppler angle
  c. low speed and small doppler angle
  d. low speed and large doppler angle
  e. more than one of the above

6.21 For disturbed or turbulent flow in Figure 6.4, (C) could represent
  a. high speed and large doppler angle
  b. high speed and small doppler angle
  c. low speed and small doppler angle
  d. low speed and large doppler angle
  e. more than one of the above

6.22 Doppler ultrasound provides information about flow conditions only at the site of measurement. True or false?

6.23 Stenosis affects
 a. peak systolic flow speed
 b. end diastolic flow speed
 c. spectral broadening
 d. window
 e. all of the above

6.24 Spectral broadening is a _____ of the spectral trace.
 a. vertical thickening
 b. horizontal thickening
 c. brightening
 d. darkening
 e. horizontal shift

6.25 If all cells in a vessel were moving at the same constant speed, the spectral trace would be a _____ line.
 a. thin horizontal
 b. thin vertical
 c. thick horizontal
 d. thick vertical
 e. none of the above

6.26 In Figure 6.8c, in which part of the flow cycle is spectral broadening (bandwidth) the least?
 a. acceleration
 b. deceleration
 c. neither

6.27 Disturbed flow produces a narrower spectrum. True or false?

6.28 Turbulent flow produces a narrower spectrum. True or false?

6.29 As stenosis is increased, which of the following increase(s)?
 a. vessel diameter
 b. systolic doppler shift
 c. diastolic doppler shift
 d. spectral broadening
 e. more than one of the above

6.30 Higher flow speed always produces a higher doppler shift on a spectral display. True or false?

6.31 Spectral broadening _____ the window.
 a. increases
 b. decreases
 c. brightens
 d. does not affect

6.32 Flow reversal in diastole indicates
 a. stenosis
 b. aneurysm

    c. high distal impedance

    d. low distal impedance

    e. more than one of the above

6.33 Decreased distal impedance normally causes end diastolic flow to

    a. increase

    b. decrease

    c. be disturbed

    d. become turbulent

    e. more than one of the above

6.34 Match the following.

_____ **a.** narrow spectra	1. small vessels
	2. large vessels
_____ **b.** broad spectra	3. medium vessels
_____ **c.** intermediate spectra	

6.35 Which is expected at the center of a vessel? Narrow or broad spectrum?

6.36 Which is expected at the center of a vessel? Higher or lower flow speeds?

6.37 Spectral broadening always indicates turbulence. True or false?

6.38 Increasing distal impedance and increasing doppler angle have the same effect on the spectral display. True or false?

6.39 Which normally has the smallest end diastolic flow?

    a. common carotid artery

    b. internal carotid artery

    c. external carotid artery

6.40 Zero and reverse flow in late diastole are normal findings in some locations of the circulation. True or false?

6.41 The pulsatility index approach works because flow impedance _____ over cardiac cycle. This is because the vessels are _____. In this case, impedance is _____ at lower pressures and _____ at higher pressures.

6.42 Under what condition can a relatively high doppler shift come from a relatively slowly moving flow?

6.43 Under what condition can a relatively low doppler shift come from a relatively rapidly moving flow?

6.44 When the spectral trace is calibrated in flow speed (cm/s), the highest flow speed shown always represents the fastest cells in the vessel. True or false?

6.45 A region of bright color on a color-flow display always indicates the highest flow speeds. True or false?

6.46 If flow speed less than 125 cm/s and doppler shift less than 4 kHz both indicate normal flow, what operating frequency is being used if the doppler angle is 60 degrees?

    a. 1 MHz

    b. 2 MHz

    c. 3 MHz

    d. 4 MHz

    e. 5 MHz

Chapter 7

Artifacts, Performance, and Safety

Several artifacts are encountered in doppler ultrasound. These are incorrect presentations of doppler flow information. The most common of these is aliasing. However, others occur, including range ambiguity, spectrum mirror image, location mirror image, speckle, and electromagnetic interference. Artifacts encountered in sonography are discussed in Section 2.4.

Several devices and methods are available to determine if doppler ultrasound instruments are operating correctly and consistently. These devices and methods are considered in three groups: (1) those that test the operation of the instrument as a whole; (2) those that measure the beams produced by transducers; and (3) those that measure the acoustic output of the instrument. Devices and methods that deal with imaging and flow measurement must be included for performance evaluation of doppler systems. System performance is important for evaluating the instrument as a diagnostic tool. Beam profiles are important when evaluating and choosing transducers. The acoustic output of an instrument is important when considering bioeffects and safety.

Risk and safety considerations are always of interest in medical diagnostic techniques. It is desirable to gain information that will be useful in guiding patient management while, at the same time, minimizing any risk

145

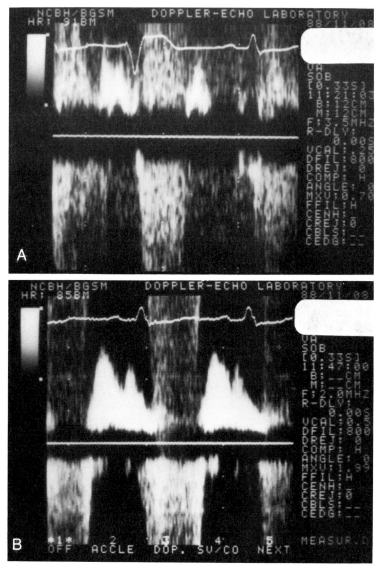

Figure 7.1. Two examples of aliasing in doppler echocardiography. (Courtesy of A. M. Nomeir.)

resulting from the diagnostic procedure. Biologic effects of ultrasound exposure have been studied in cells, plants, and experimental animals and several epidemiologic studies have been performed. From this information we develop an approach to the appropriate and prudent use of doppler ultrasound as a medical diagnostic tool.

7.1
Artifacts

Aliasing is the most common artifact encountered in doppler ultra-sound. There is an upper limit to doppler shift that can be detected by pulsed instruments. If the doppler shift frequency exceeds one half the pulse repetition frequency (normally in the 5 to 30 kHz range), aliasing occurs (Fig. 7.1).[54] Improper doppler shift information (improper direction and improper value) results. An analogous optical form of aliasing occurs in motion pictures when wagon wheels appear to rotate at various speeds and in reverse direction. Higher pulse repetition frequencies (Table 7.1) permit higher doppler shifts to be detected but also increase the chance of the range ambiguity artifact (discussed later in this section). Continuous-wave doppler instruments do not have this limitation (but neither do they provide depth selectivity).

Color Plate V illustrates aliasing with color flow doppler. Figure 7.2 illustrates aliasing in the popliteal artery of a normal subject. This figure also illustrates how aliasing can be eliminated (Table 7.2) by increasing pulse repetition frequency, increasing doppler angle (which decreases the doppler shift for a given flow), or by baseline shifting. The latter is an electronic "cut and paste" technique that moves the misplaced aliasing peaks over to their proper location. It is a successful technique as long as there are no legitimate doppler shifts in the region of the aliasing. If there are, they will get moved over to an inappropriate location along with the aliasing peaks. (This would happen if the baseline were shifted further down in Figure 7.2e.) Other approaches to eliminating aliasing include

Table 7.1
Aliasing and Range-Ambiguity Artifact Values

Pulse Repetition Frequency (kHz)	Doppler Shift Above Which Aliasing Occurs (kHz)	Range Beyond Which Ambiguity Occurs (cm)
5.0	2.5	15
7.5	3.7	10
10.0	5.0	7
12.5	6.2	6
15.0	7.5	5
17.5	8.7	4
20.0	10.0	3
25.0	12.5	3
30.0	15.0	2

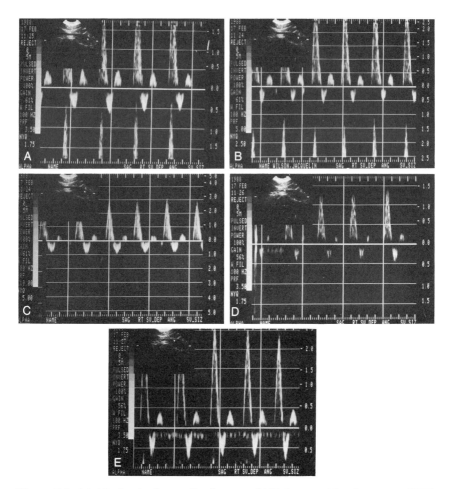

Figure 7.2. (a) Aliasing in the popliteal artery. (b) Pulse repetition frequency (PRF) is increased. (c) PRF is increased again. (d) Doppler angle is increased. (e) Baseline is shifted down to reduce or eliminate aliasing. (From Taylor KJW, Burns PN, Wells PNT (eds): Clinical Applications of Doppler Ultrasound. New York, Raven Press, 1988. Reprinted with permission; courtesy of K. J. W. Taylor.)

changing to a lower frequency doppler transducer or changing to a continuous-wave instrument.

Aliasing occurs with the pulsed system because it is a sampling system. That is, a pulsed system acquires samples of the desired doppler shift frequency from which it must be synthesized. If samples are taken often enough, the correct result is achieved. Figure 7.3 shows sampling of a sig-

Table 7.2
Methods of Reducing or Eliminating Aliasing

1. Increase pulse repetition frequency.
2. Increase doppler angle.
3. Shift the baseline.
4. Lower the operating frequency.
5. Use a continuous-wave device.

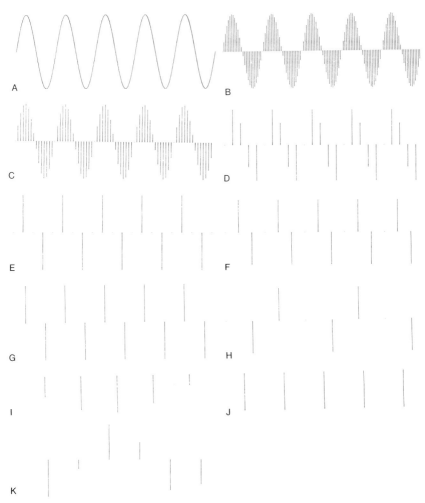

Figure 7.3. Sample of (a) a 5-cycle voltage; (b) 25 samples per cycle; (c) 15 samples per cycle; (d) 5 samples per cycle; (e) 4 samples per cycle; (f) 3 samples per cycle; (g) 2 samples per cycle; (h) 1 sample per cycle; (i) 1 sample per cycle; (j) 1 sample per cycle; (k) 1 sample per cycle. In the last four cases, aliasing occurs.

nal. Sufficient sampling yields the correct result. Insufficient sampling yields an incorrect result. This is also illustrated in Figure 7.4.

The nyquist limit or nyquist frequency describes the minimum number of samples required to avoid aliasing. There must be at least two samples per cycle of the desired wave in order for it to be obtained correctly. For a complicated signal such as a doppler signal containing many frequencies (see Fig. 6.1), the sampling rate must be such that at least two samples occur for each cycle of the highest frequency present. To restate this rule, if the highest doppler shift frequency present in a signal exceeds one half the pulse repetition frequency, aliasing will occur (Fig. 7.5).

In an attempt to solve the aliasing problem by increasing pulse repetition frequency, the range ambiguity[55-57] problem can be encountered. This occurs when a pulse is emitted before all the echoes from the previous pulse have been received. When this happens, early echoes from the last pulse are simultaneously received with late echoes from the previous pulse. This causes difficulty with the ranging process described in Sections 2.1 and 5.2. The instrument is unable to determine whether an echo is an

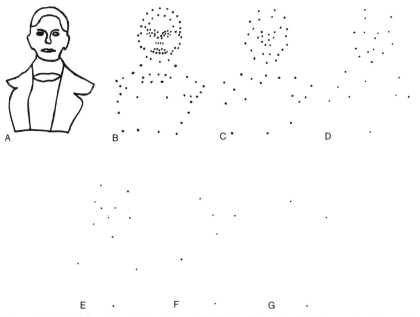

Figure 7.4. (a) A free-hand drawing of Christian Doppler. (b) 96 samples from (a), (c) 48 samples, (d) 24 samples, (e) 12 samples, (f) 6 samples, (g) 3 samples. In the last three cases, connecting the dots would yield an image that would bear no resemblance to (a). Indeed, in (g), a triangle would result. These cases are undersampled, yielding an "aliased" result.

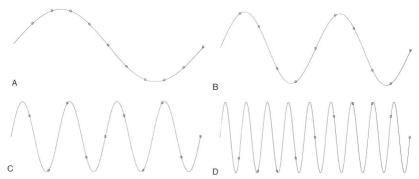

Figure 7.5. Signal voltages sampled at 10 points (o). (a) 1 cycle; (b) 2 cycles; (c) 4 cycles; (d) 9 cycles. As signal frequency is increased, aliasing occurs when the nyquist limit is exceeded (in this case beyond 5 cycles). Thus, (d) is aliasing. It can be seen that connecting the o's with a smooth curve would yield a 1-cycle representation of what is actually a 9-cycle signal voltage.

early one (superficial) from the last pulse or a late one (deep) from the previous pulse (Fig. 7.6). To avoid this difficulty it simply assumes that all echoes are derived from the last pulse and that these echoes have originated from some depth as determined by the 13 μs/cm rule (see Section 2.1). As long as all echoes are received before the next pulse is sent out, this will be true. However, with high pulse repetition frequencies, this may not be the case. Doppler flow information may, therefore, come from locations other than the assumed one (the gate location). In effect, multiple gates or sample volumes are operating at different depths. Table 7.1 lists, for various pulse repetition frequencies, the ranges beyond which ambiguity occurs. Table 7.3 lists, for various depths, the maximum doppler shift frequency that will avoid aliasing and the range ambiguity problem. Maximum flow speeds for given angles are also listed. Instruments often increase pulse repetition frequency (to avoid aliasing) into the range where range ambiguity occurs. Multiple sample gates are shown on the display to indicate this condition. An approximate relationship between maximum flow speed and maximum depth to avoid both aliasing and range ambiguity is as follows:

$$\text{maximum flow speed (cm/s)} = \frac{3000}{\text{maximum depth (cm)} \times \text{frequency} \times \text{cosine doppler angle}}$$

$$v_m = \frac{3000}{d_m f \cos \theta}$$

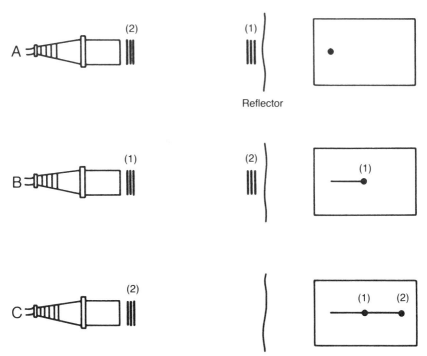

Figure 7.6. Ambiguity caused by sending out a pulse before a reflection from the previous pulse is received. (a) A pulse (2) is sent out just as a previous pulse (1) is reflected. (b) The spot begins to move across the display. The first reflection arrives at the transducer when the second pulse reflects. (c) The second reflection arrives at the transducer, putting a bright spot (2) on the display at the position corresponding to the reflector. The spot (1) in the center of the display resulting from the arrival of the earlier pulse indicates a reflector at a location where there is none. (d) Transvaginal image shows the pulsed doppler range gate (arrow) set at 33 mm within an ovary. (e) The resulting doppler spectrum shows a waveform typical of the external iliac artery. (f) An identical signal was obtained when the range was increased to 63 mm, proving that the signal actually originated from the external iliac artery at this depth. (g) A strong arterial doppler signal was obtained in this examination when the range gate (arrow) was placed within the urinary bladder at a depth of 31 mm. (h) An identical signal was detected when the range gate depth was increased to 61 mm, indicating that the signal actually arose from an artery at this depth. (i) With the range gate (arrow) placed at a depth of 50 mm in the uterus of a pregnant woman, 16 weeks' gestation, signals (j) typical of the external iliac artery were detected. (k) Slight adjustment of the range gate (arrow) produced the desired umbilical artery signal (l), eliminating the artifactual iliac artery signal caused by range ambiguity. (d through l from Gill RW, Kossoff MB, Kossoff G, Griffiths KA: New class of pulsed doppler US ambiguity at short ranges. Radiology 173:272, 1989.)

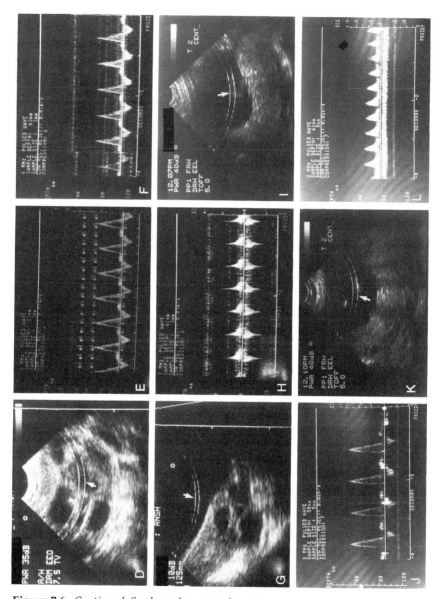

Figure 7.6. *Continued. See legend on opposite page*

Table 7.3
Aliasing and Range-Ambiguity Limits

Depth (cm)	PRF (kHz)	Nyquist Limit (kHz)	Maximum Flow Speed (cm/s)		
			0	30	60
1	77.0	38.0	585	673	1170
2	38.0	19.0	293	336	585
4	19.0	10.0	146	168	293
8	10.0	4.8	73	84	146
16	4.8	2.4	37	42	73

For various depths, the maximum pulse-reception frequency (PRF) that avoids range ambiguity and the maximum doppler shift frequency (nyquist limit) that avoids aliasing are listed. Maximum flow speeds corresponding to the maximum doppler shift are also listed for three doppler angles (degrees) assuming 5-MHz operating frequency.

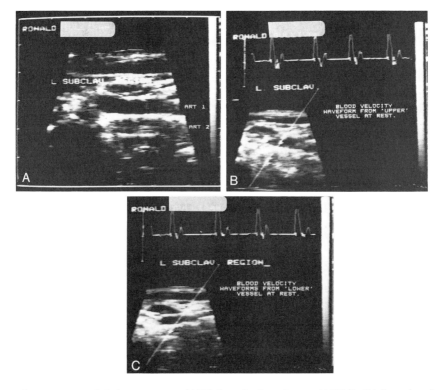

Figure 7.7. (a) Subclavian artery (ART 1) and mirror image (ART 2); (b) flow signal from artery; (c) flow signal from mirror image. (Courtesy of T. N. Needham.)

Range ambiguity in color-flow doppler, as in sonography, places echoes (color doppler shifts in this case) that have come from deep locations after a subsequent pulse was emitted in shallow locations where they do not belong.

The mirror image artifact described in Section 2.4 can also occur with doppler systems. This means that an image of a vessel and a source of doppler shifted echoes can be duplicated on the opposite side of a strong reflector (such as a bone). The duplicated vessel containing flow could be misinterpreted as an additional vessel. It will have a spectrum similar to that for the real vessel. Figure 7.7 shows an example of image and spectrum duplication of the subclavian artery. The strong reflector in this case may be the pleura.

A mirror image of a doppler spectrum can appear on the opposite side of the baseline when, indeed, flow is unidirectional and should appear only on one side of the baseline. This is an electronic duplication of the spectral information. It can occur when receiver gain is set too high (causing overloading in the receiver and cross talk between the two flow channels) or with low gain (where the receiver has difficulty determining the sign of the doppler shift). It can also occur when doppler angle is near 90 degrees (Fig. 7.8a,b). Here the duplication is usually legitimate. This is because beams are focused and not cylindrical in shape. Thus, portions of the beam can experience flow toward while other portions can experience flow away (Fig. 7.8c).

Doppler spectra have a speckle quality to them similar to that observed in sonography. Speckle is a result of interference effects of scattered sound from the distribution of scatterers (erythrocytes) in the blood. Because the ultrasound pulse encounters several scatterers at any point in its travel, several echoes are generated simultaneously. These may arrive at the transducer in such a way that they re-enforce (constructive interference) or partially or totally cancel (destructive interference) each other. This results in a displayed dot pattern that does not directly represent individual scatterers but rather represents an interference pattern of the scatterer distribution scanned. This phenomenon is called acoustic speckle. It is analogous to the speckle phenomenon observed when a laser is shone on a wall.

Occasionally, a spectral trace can show a straight line adjacent to and parallel to the baseline, often on both sides as in Figure 7.9. Apparently, this is due to 60-Hz interference from power lines or power supply. It can make determination of low or absent diastolic flow difficult. Electromagnetic interference from power lines and nearby equipment can also cloud the spectral display with lines or "snow."

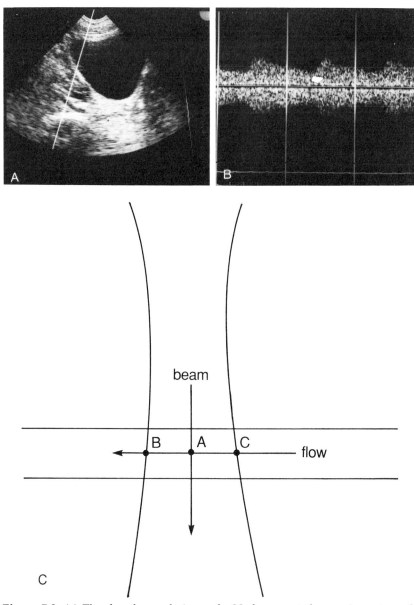

Figure 7.8. (a) The doppler angle is nearly 90 degrees at the ovarian artery. (b) Spectral mirror image with low-impedance flow on both sides of the baseline. (c) Because beams are focused and not cylindrical in shape, portions of the beam (C) can experience flow toward while other portions (B) can experience flow away when the beam axis intersects (A) the flow at 90 degrees. (a and b from Taylor KJW, Holland S: Doppler ultrasound I. Basic principles, instrumentation and pitfalls. Radiology 174:297–307, 1990.)

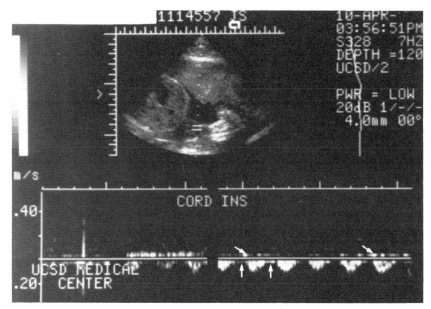

Figure 7.9. Sixty-hertz interference (arrows) above and below the baseline. (Courtesy of D. H. Pretorius.)

7.2
Performance

Tissue- and blood-mimicking phantoms are commercially available for the evaluation of doppler instruments (Figs. 7.10 and 7.11). These are useful for testing the effective penetration of the doppler beam, the ability to discriminate between different flow directions, accuracy of sample volume location, and accuracy of the measured flow speed.[58] Doppler flow phantoms fall into two groups: those that use a blood-mimicking liquid (e.g., Sephadex in water, polystyrene microspheres suspended in a water and glycerol mixture, mixture of water and machine-cutting oil, and aqueous starch suspensions) and those that use a moving string for scattering the ultrasound.[59] The latter can be calibrated more easily and can produce pulsatile and reverse motions (Fig. 7.11b). The former have some difficulties, such as the presence of bubbles and nonuniform flow, but can be arranged to more easily simulate clinical conditions, such as tissue attenuation.[58] They can be calibrated with an electromagnetic flowmeter or by volume collection over time.

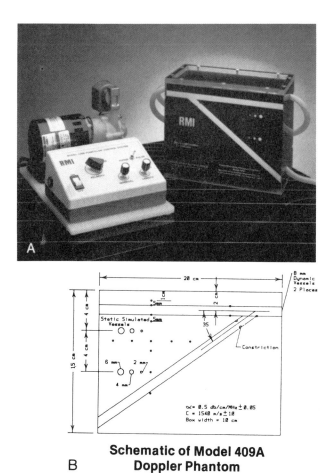

Schematic of Model 409A
B   Doppler Phantom

Figure 7.10. Commercial doppler phantom and flow system. (Courtesy of Radiation Measurements, Inc.)

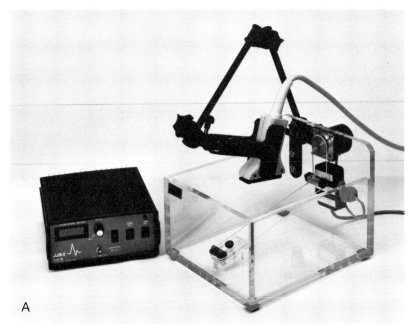

A

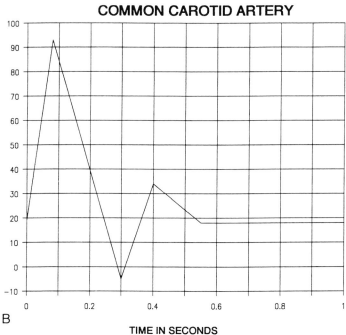

COMMON CAROTID ARTERY

B

TIME IN SECONDS

Figure 7.11. (a) Moving string phantom and controller. (b) Example of string speed versus time. (Courtesy of JJ&A Instruments.)

Imaging performance in duplex and color-flow instruments is determined by measuring the following parameters:

1. system sensitivity and dynamic range
2. contrast resolution (Section 2.3)
3. detail resolution (Section 2.2)
4. dead zone
5. range (depth or distance) accuracy (Sections 2.1 and 2.3)
6. compensation (swept gain) operation (Section 2.3)

These may all be measured using the 100-mm test object of the American Institute of Ultrasound in Medicine (AIUM) (Fig. 7.12). This test object is composed of a series of 0.75-mm diameter stainless-steel rods arranged in a pattern between two transparent plastic sides. The other sides are made of thin acrylic plastic sheets on which the transducer may be placed using a coupling medium. The tank is filled with a mixture of alcohol, algae inhibitor, and water that has a propagation speed of 1.54 mm/μs at room temperature. The speed varies by less than 1 percent when the temperature is changed by 5°C. Therefore, results with this test object are relatively insensitive to normal fluctuations in room temperature. Construction details and procedures for its use have been published.[60,61] These test objects are available commercially (Fig. 7.13).

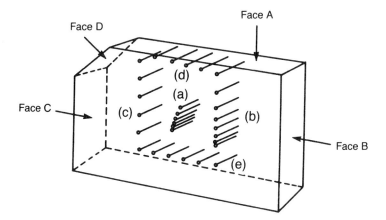

Figure 7.12. The AIUM 100-mm test object. Rod groups are used for measuring (a) axial resolution; (b) or (c) lateral resolution; (c) range accuracy and receiver compensation; (d) dead zone; and (a) through (e) registration accuracy. Any rod imaged may be used for sensitivity or dynamic range measurements.

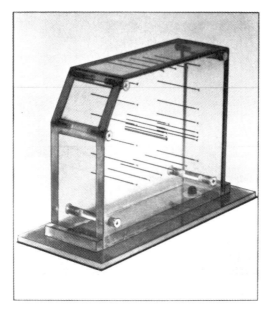

version of the AIUM test object. (Courtesy

To obtain consistent measurements of axial and lateral resolution and dead zone, even with a given transducer and diagnostic instrument, it is necessary to perform the test at consistent control settings. Usually, it is best to measure relative system sensitivity first and then increase the sensitivity settings a fixed amount for performing the other tests.

Relative system sensitivity is a measure of how weak a reflection an instrument can display. It is obtained by finding the gain or attenuation setting (with no compensation) at which a particular rod in the test object produces a barely discernible display. Any imaged rod may be chosen for this measurement. Usually, the top rod in group (a) or the bottom rod in group (c) is used for system sensitivity measurements (Fig. 7.12). For the remaining measurements, 10 dB are added to the system sensitivity settings required to barely display the chosen rod.

Axial resolution is measured with rod group (a). The transducer is placed on face A above the rod group. Not all the rods will be seen separately on the display. The spacing of the two closest rods in the group that are seen separately on the display is equal to the axial resolution (Fig. 7.14). Axial resolution measured with the test object usually does not reflect the best possible resolution of the diagnostic system. The measure-

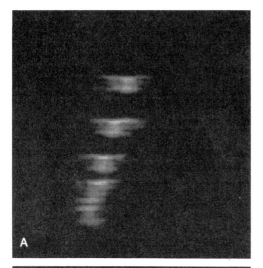

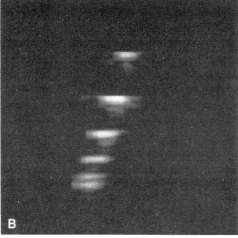

Figure 7.14. (a) An image of a set of six rods in the AIUM Test Object (Section 7.2). They are separated by 5, 4, 3, 2, and 1 mm from top to bottom. This scan was made using a transducer that produces 3.5-MHz ultrasound. The first three rods have been separated, whereas the images of the last three rods have merged; therefore, the axial resolution is about 3 mm. This image also shows small reverberation echoes behind each image. (b) The same rods imaged with a 5-MHz transducer. Higher frequency transducers produce shorter pulse lengths and therefore provide improved axial resolution.

ment, however, is a consistency check for use with a given transducer and instrument.

Lateral resolution is measured with rod group (b). The transducer is scanned along face B. Not all the rods will be seen separately on the display. The spacing of the two closest rods in the group that are seen separately on the display is equal to the lateral resolution (Fig. 7.15a). Lateral resolution at a range from 1 to 11 cm can be determined by measuring the width of the line representing each rod in group (c) after the transducer is scanned across face A of the test object (Fig. 7.15b).

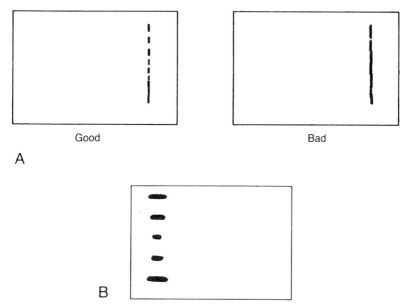

Figure 7.15. Lateral resolution. (a) Using rod group (b) in Figure 7.12, separations from 3 to 25 mm may be viewed. On the left, lateral resolution is about 5 mm. On the right, it is about 25 mm. (b) Using rod group (c) in Figure 7.12, the widths of rod images at various depths give lateral resolutions at these depths. A segmented picture of the beam is also presented with this view.

The dead zone is the distance closest to the transducer in which imaging cannot be performed. It is measured with rod group (d). The transducer is scanned across face A. The distance from the transducer to the first rod imaged is equal to the dead zone.

Range accuracy is measured with rod group (c). The rods should appear on the display at 1, 3, 5, 7, 9, and 11 cm from the transducer (Fig. 7.16). Relative distances between the rods should be accurate to at least 2 mm or less. The space between the rods at 1 and 11 cm should be recorded with calipers and then measured with marker dots placed parallel to rod group (e). If this indicates that the distance between the rods at 1 and 11 cm differs from the true 10 cm by more than 2 mm, then the horizontal and vertical display scales are not identical.

Compensation operation is measured using rod group (c). The transducer is placed on face A above this rod group. With no compensation, the attenuator or gain settings required to display each rod at a given gray level are recorded. This is then done again with compensation on. The

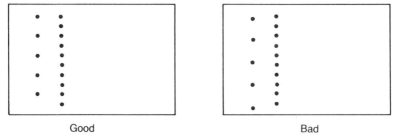

Good   Bad

Figure 7.16. Range accuracy is tested using rod group (c) in Figure 7.12. The rods should appear with 2-cm separations as on the left. One-centimeter marker dots are displayed here as well.

difference between the settings for each rod as a function of distance is the compensation characteristic.

The gray-scale dynamic range is the difference between gain or attenuator settings (dB) that produce (1) barely discernible and (2) maximum brightness displays for the same reflection. Any rod imaged may be chosen for this measurement.

Several other objects are available commercially for testing imaging performance. These fall into two categories: test objects (e.g., the AIUM test object discussed earlier) and tissue-equivalent phantoms. Tissue-

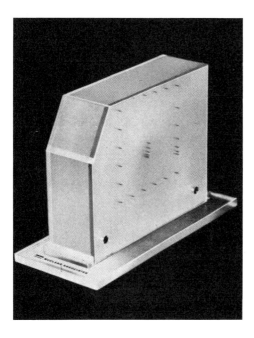

Figure 7.17. AIUM test object filled with tissue-equivalent material. (Courtesy of Nuclear Associates.)

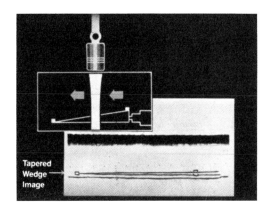

Figure 7.18. A commercial version of the SUAR test object. (Courtesy of Nuclear Associates.)

equivalent phantoms have some characteristics representative of tissues (e.g., scattering or attenuation properties), whereas test objects do not. Some objects are combinations of the two (e.g., an AIUM test object filled with tissue-equivalent medium rather than a water-alcohol mixture) (Fig. 7.17). The sensitivity, uniformity, and axial resolution (SUAR) test object

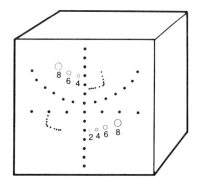

Figure 7.19. Commercial tissue-equivalent phantom containing wires and echo-free (cystic) areas. (Courtesy of ATS Laboratories.)

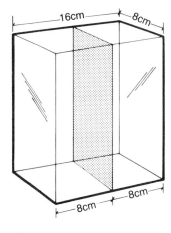

Model 508

Figure 7.20. Commerical version of beam-profile test object. (Courtesy of ATS Laboratories.) Scans with such a test object are shown in Figures 2.30b and 2.31b.

uses a wedge cavity in a block to allow axial resolution measurement over a continuous range of separations (Fig. 7.18). Tissue-equivalent phantoms containing echo-free (cystic) regions (Fig. 7.19), scattering layers for scattered beam profile visualization (see Figs. 2.30b, 2.31b, and 7.20), arrays of echo-free cylinders of various radii at various depths (see Figs. 2.30a, 2.31a, and 7.21), cones and cylinders containing materials of various scattering strengths (Fig. 7.22), or blocks of various scattering materials (gray-

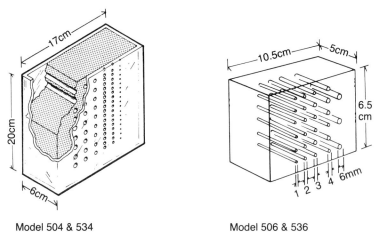

Model 504 & 534   Model 506 & 536

Figure 7.21. Commercial versions of resolution-penetration phantoms. (Courtesy of ATS Laboratories.) Scans with such a test object are shown in Figures 2.30a and 2.31a.

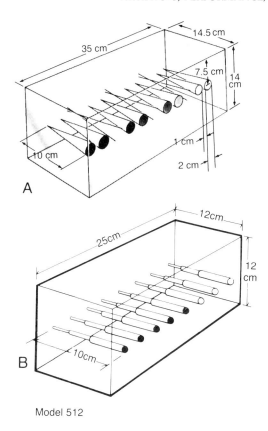

A

B

Model 512

Figure 7.22. Commercial versions of contrast/detail resolution phantoms. (a) Courtesy of Nuclear Associates; (b) courtesy of ATS Laboratories.

scale levels) are available (Fig. 7.23). The particle-image resolution test object (PIRTO) is filled with polystyrene spheres randomly distributed in a low-attenuation, low-scatter gel (Fig. 7.24).

The AIUM test object described in this section measures one beam parameter, the beam diameter, which is equal to lateral resolution. How-

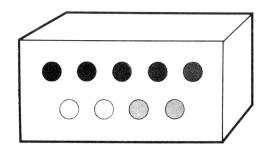

Figure 7.23. Commercial version of gray-scale test phantom. (Courtesy of ATS Laboratories.)

Model 531

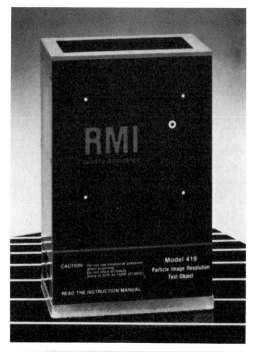

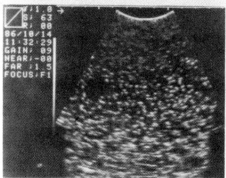

Figure 7.24. Commercial version of a PIRTO phantom. (Courtesy of Radiation Measurements, Inc.)

ever, it does this only at one distance from the transducer: the distance from face B to rod group (b) in Figure 7.12. The use of rod group (c) in Figure 7.12 does not suffer from this same restriction. However, there is some distortion of the lateral resolution measurements in rod group (c) because of shadowing of lower rods by rods in the focal region. The test object is used to make this measurement using the ultrasound imaging instrument as a whole (the rod reflections are imaged on the instrument display). Scattering-layer test objects (see Figs. 2.30b, 2.31b, and 7.20) pro-

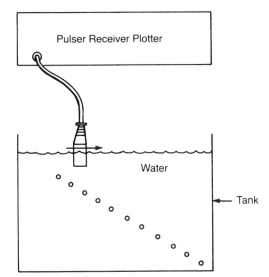

Figure 7.25. A beam profiler consists of a pulser, receiver, plotter, transducer, and tank with rods at various distances from the transducer. The transducer is scanned over the rods.

vide qualitative beam presentations. A beam profiler is a device designed to give three-dimensional (quantitative) reflection amplitude information. It uses rods at various distances from the transducer (Fig. 7.25). The transducer is pulsed as it is scanned across the tank. Reflections are received from each rod, and voltage amplitude is measured. As the sound beam passes over a rod, the reflected amplitude increases, goes through a maximum, and then decreases. Then, the next rod (at a greater distance) is

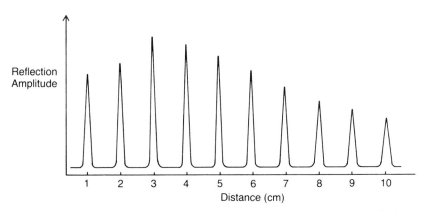

Figure 7.26. Beam profile plotted by the system in Figure 7.25. Each peak shows reflection amplitude as scanned across the rod that is at the distance indicated from the transducer. The amplitude is maximum at the near-zone length of an unfocused transducer or at the focal region of a focused transducer (Section 2.2).

encountered with a similar reflection behavior. This continues until all rods have been encountered. A beam profile can be plotted from this procedure (Fig. 7.26). A beam profile does not actually give a profile of a beam (i.e., it does not plot acoustic amplitude or intensity across the beam at several distances from the transducer as it appears to do). It actually plots reflection amplitude received at the transducer, and it could be called a reflection profiler. For imaging instruments, however, this profile is a useful thing. Such profiles are often supplied with transducers to show beam characteristics obtained by this method. Hydrophones (discussed later in this section) can also be beam profilers in that they can measure pressure and intensity distributions across beams (Figs. 7.27 and 7.28).

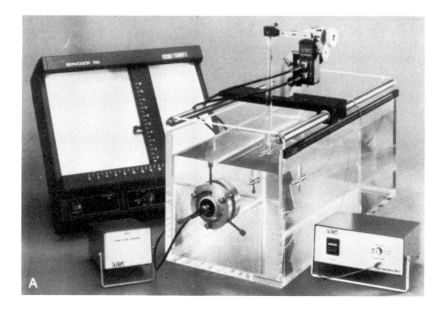

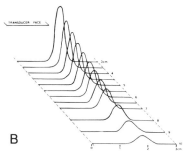

Figure 7.27. (a) Hydrophone system for measuring (b) beam profile. (Courtesy of Medisonics.)

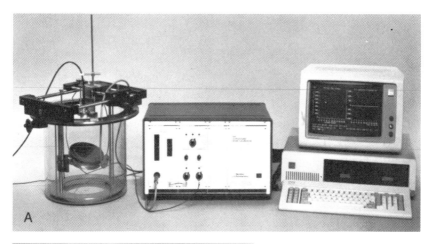

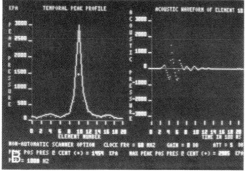

Figure 7.28. (a) Linear array membrane hydrophone system for measuring (b) beam profile. (Courtesy of Nuclear Enterprises.)

Pulses produced by ultrasound transducers contain a range of frequencies called the bandwidth. Transducer specifications often include a picture of the frequency spectrum of the pulses produced. This is a plot of amplitude (of each frequency component) versus frequency (Fig. 7.29). It is obtained by receiving the pulse with a hydrophone or with the same transducer that produced it (after reflection from a sphere, rod, or plate). The electric pulse from the hydrophone or transducer is sent to a spectrum analyzer, which breaks it down into its component frequencies and displays them.

Several devices can measure the acoustic output of ultrasound imaging instruments. Only one, the hydrophone, will be discussed here. The hydrophone is a small (1 mm in diameter or less) transducer element mounted on the end of a narrow tube or hollow needle (Fig. 7.30). Its size causes it to receive sound reasonably well from all directions without altering the sound by its presence. In response to the varying pressure of the

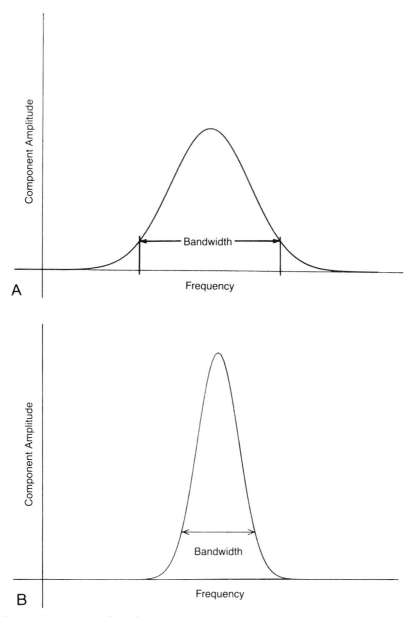

Figure 7.29. A plot of the frequencies present in an ultrasound pulse. Component amplitude is the amplitude of each frequency component present. Bandwidth is the frequency range within which the amplitudes exceed some reference value. Plot (a) represents a broad band, low quality factor, damped pulse. Plot (b) represents a narrow band, high quality factor, undamped pulse.

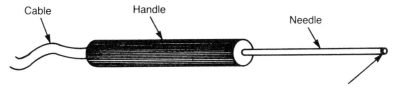

Figure 7.30. A hydrophone consists of a small transducer element mounted on the end of a needle.

sound, it produces a varying voltage that can be displayed on an oscillo-scope. A picture similar to that in Figure 7.28 is produced, from which frequency, pulse repetition frequency, and duty factor can be calculated. If the hydrophone calibration is known (relationship between voltage pro-duced and pressure applied), pressure amplitude may also be determined.

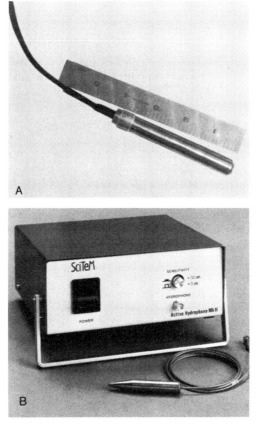

Figure 7.31. Commercial hydrophones. (a) Courtesy of Nuclear Associates; (b) courtesy of Medisonics.

If propagation speed is known, wavelength and spatial pulse length can be calculated (see Section 2.1). If impedance is known, intensity can be calculated. Hydrophones are available commercially (Fig. 7.31) and are relatively inexpensive and simple to use. Polyvinylidene fluoride (PVDF) is the thin film material commonly used in modern hydrophones.

7.3
Bioeffects

In any diagnostic test, there may be some risk (some probability of damage or injury). For diagnostic ultrasound, the sonologist and sonographer need to know something about this risk. Risk can be weighed against benefit to determine the appropriateness of the diagnostic procedure (Fig. 7.32). Knowledge of how to minimize the risk is useful to everyone involved in diagnostic ultrasound.

There are several sources of bioeffects information (Fig. 7.33). However, a complete knowledge of the bioeffects of ultrasound is unavailable. What types of injury can diagnostic ultrasound produce in patients? Under what conditions?

The biologic effects of ultrasound have been studied for about 60 years. Numerous reports dealing with mechanisms, effects on cells, effects on experimental plants and animals, and epidemiology have appeared in the scientific and medical literature.[62-71] Tables 7.4 to 7.10 present several official statements of the American Institute of Ultrasound in Medicine (AIUM) regarding thermal mechanism, cavitation, epidemiology, in vivo mammalian bioeffects, clinical safety, safety in training and research, and in vitro biologic effects. This represents a 12-year history of the AIUM in developing and disseminating official statements dealing with bioeffects

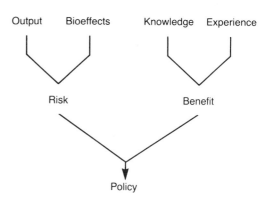

Figure 7.32. Ultrasound risk and benefit information. Risk information comes from experimental bioeffects, epidemiology, and instrument output data. Benefit information comes from knowledge and experience in ultrasound imaging use and efficacy. Together they lead to policy on the prudent use of ultrasound imaging in medicine.

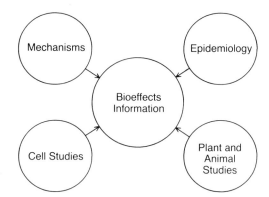

Figure 7.33. Bioeffects information sources.

and safety of diagnostic ultrasound. The first statement was the AIUM statement on mammalian in vivo biologic effects of August 1976. It was revised in 1978 and reaffirmed in 1982. It was revised in 1987, the same year in which four groups of other statements were approved. Other statements initially approved in 1982 and 1983 were revised in 1988. All of these are included in the tables.

Table 7.4
Conclusions Regarding a Thermal Bioeffects Mechanism
(Approved October 1987)

1. A thermal criterion is one reasonable approach to specifying potentially hazardous exposures for diagnostic ultrasound.
2. Based solely on a thermal criterion, a diagnostic exposure that produces a maximum temperature rise of 1°C above normal physiological levels may be used without reservation in clinical examinations.
3. An *in situ* temperature rise to or above 41°C is considered hazardous in fetal exposures; the longer this temperature elevation is maintained, the greater is the likelihood for damage to occur.
4. Analytical models of ultrasonically induced heating have been applied successfully to *in vivo* mammalian situations. In those clinical situations where local tissue temperatures are not measured, estimates of temperature elevations can be made by employing such analytical models.
5. Calculations of ultrasonically induced temperature elevation, based on a simplified tissue model and a simplified model of stationary beams, suggest the following. For examinations of fetal soft tissues with typical perfusion rates, employing center frequencies between 2 and 10 MHz and beam widths* less than 11 wavelengths, the computed temperature rise will not be significantly above 1°C if the *in situ* SATA intensity† does not exceed 200 mW/cm². If the beam width does not exceed eight wavelengths the corresponding intensity is 300 mW/cm². However, if the same beam impinges on fetal bone, the local temperature rise may be much higher.

*−6 dB beam width, according to AIUM/NEMA definition.
†SATA intensity refers to the spatial average value over the focal area.
(From AIUM: Bioeffects considerations for the safety of diagnostic ultrasound. J Ultrasound Med 7(9): Supplement, 1988. Reprinted with permission.)

Table 7.5
Conclusions Regarding Cavitation
(Approved October 1987)

1. Acoustic cavitation may occur with short pulses and has the potential for producing deleterious biological effects.
2. Currently available information indicates that pulses with peak pressures greater than 10 MPa (3300 W/cm²) can induce cavitation in mammals.*
3. With the limited data available, it is not possible to specify *threshold* pressure amplitudes at which acoustic cavitation will occur in mammals, with diagnostically relevant pulse lengths and repetition rates.

*Evidence from observations with lithotripters.
(From AIUM: Bioeffects considerations for the safety of diagnostic ultrasound. J Ultrasound Med 7(9): Supplement, 1988. Reprinted with permission.)

Table 7.6
Conclusions Regarding Epidemiology
(Approved October 1987)

1. Widespread clinical use over 25 years has not established any adverse effect arising from exposure to diagnostic ultrasound.
2. Randomized clinical studies are the most rigorous method for assessing potential adverse effects of diagnostic ultrasound. Studies using this methodology show no evidence of an effect on birthweight in humans.*
3. Other epidemiologic studies have shown no causal association of diagnostic ultrasound with any of the adverse fetal outcomes studied.*

*The acoustic exposure levels in these studies may not be representativeof the full range of current fetal exposures.
(From AIUM: Bioeffects considerations for the safety of diagnostic ultrasound. J Ultrasound Med 7(9): Supplement, 1988. Reprinted with permission.)

Table 7.7
Conclusions Regarding In Vivo Mammalian Bioeffects
(Approved October 1987)

A review of bioeffects data supports the following statement as an update of the AIUM Statement on In Vivo Mammalian Bioeffects:
In the low megahertz frequency range there have been (as of this date) no independently confirmed significant biological effects in mammalian tissue exposed *in vivo* to unfocused ultrasound with intensities* below 100 mW/cm², or to focused† ultrasound with intensities below 1 W/cm². Furthermore, for exposure times‡ greater than 1 second and less than 500 seconds for unfocused ultrasound or 50 seconds for focused ultrasound, such effects have not been demonstrated even at higher intensities, when the product of intensity and exposure time is less than 50 joules/cm².

*Free-field spatial peak, temporal average (SPTA) for continuous wave exposures, and for pulsed-mode exposures with pulses repeated at a frequency greater than 100 Hz.
†Quarter-power (−6 dB) beam width smaller than four wavelengths or 4 mm, whichever is less at the exposure frequency.
‡Total time including off-time as well as on-time for repeated pulse exposures.
(From AIUM: Bioeffects considerations for the safety of diagnostic ultrasound. J Ultrasound Med 7(9): Supplement, 1988. Reprinted with permission.)

Table 7.8
American Institute of Ultrasound in Medicine Official Statement on Clinical Safety
(Approved October 1982; Revised and Approved March 1988)

Diagnostic ultrasound has been in use since the late 1950s. Given its known benefits and recognized efficacy for medical diagnosis, including use during human pregnancy, the American Institute of Ultrasound in Medicine herein addresses the clinical safety of such use:

No confirmed biological effects on patients or instrument operators caused by exposure at intensities typical of present diagnostic ultrasound instruments have ever been reported. Although the possibility exists that such biological effects may be identified in the future, current data indicate that the benefits to patients of the prudent use of diagnostic ultrasound outweigh the risks, if any, that may be present.

(From AIUM: Bioeffects considerations for the safety of diagnostic ultrasound. J Ultrasound Med 7(9): Supplement, 1988. Reprinted with permission.)

To this author's knowledge no specific studies have been performed with regard to bioeffects of doppler ultrasound. This is because doppler ultrasound is not fundamentally different from imaging ultrasound. Ultrasound beams of similar frequencies are used in both applications. It is primarily the signal processing done in the receiver that is different between the two systems. However, continuous-wave sound is used in some doppler applications and, in pulsed-wave doppler, longer pulses (typically 5 to 30 cycles) and higher pulse repetition frequencies are commonly used yielding higher duty factors than in sonography. Thus, although higher SPPA intensities do not seem to characterize pulsed doppler, relatively high values of SPTA intensities are found with doppler instruments.[8,64]

Table 7.9
American Institute of Ultrasound in Medicine Official Statement on Safety in Training and Research
(Approved March 1983; Revised and Approved March 1988)

Diagnostic ultrasound has been in use since the late 1950s. No confirmed adverse biological effects on patients resulting from this usage have ever been reported. Although no hazard has been identified that would preclude the prudent and conservative use of diagnostic ultrasound in education and research, experience from normal diagnostic practice may or may not be relevant to extended exposure times and altered exposure conditions. It is therefore considered appropriate to make the following recommendation:

In those special situations in which examinations are to be carried out for purposes other than direct medical benefit to the individual being examined, the subject should be informed of the anticipated exposure conditions, and of how these compare with conditions for normal diagnostic practice.

(From AIUM: Bioeffects considerations for the safety of diagnostic ultrasound. J Ultrasound Med 7(9): Supplement, 1988. Reprinted with permission.)

Table 7.10
American Institute of Ultrasound in Medicine Official Statement on In Vitro
Biological Effects
(Approved October 1982; Revised and Approved March 1988)

It is difficult to evalute reports of ultrasonically induced *in vitro* biological effects with
respect to their clinical significance. The predominant physical and biological interactions
and mechanisms involved in an *in vitro* effect may not pertain to the *in vivo* situation.
Nevertheless, an *in vitro* effect must be regarded as a real biological effect.

Results from *in vitro* experiments suggest new endpoints and serve as a basis for design of
in vivo experiments. *In vitro* studies provide the capability to control experimental variables
and thus offer a means to explore and evaluate specific mechanisms. Although they may
have limited applicability to *in vivo* biological effects, such studies can disclose
fundamental intercellular or intracellular interactions.

While it is valid for authors to place their results in context and to suggest further relevant
investigations, reports of *in vitro* studies which claim direct clinical significance should be
viewed with caution.

(From AIUM: Bioeffects considerations for the safety of diagnostic ultrasound. J Ultrasound
Med 7(9): Supplement, 1988. Reprinted with permission.)

Two mechanisms of action by which ultrasound can produce biologic
effects have been considered dominant. They are absorption heating and
cavitation. Any bioeffect that can be produced by temperature rise, of
course, could be produced by ultrasound heating. Calculations based on a
thermal model of tissues have yielded the 200 and 300 mW/cm^2 SATA
intensity values shown in Table 7.4 for a 1°C temperature increase. Cavitation is known to occur with extremely high intensity pulses produced
by lithotripters. This information is summarized in Table 7.5. Currently,
there are no experimental data indicating that cavitation occurs in tissues
under the influence of diagnostic frequencies, intensities, pulse durations,
and pulse repetition frequencies.

Studies in cell culture and cell suspensions have yielded reports
regarding altered endpoints under the influence of ultrasound. In most
cases they appear to be due to cavitation, which is more likely to happen
in liquid systems than in tissues. Recently, the most active area of investigation has been sister chromatid exchange (SCE).[64] Variable, inconclu-
sive, and irreproducible results in this area have made it impossible to
derive conclusions or recommendations or use this approach as a basis for
risk assessment.[63,64,71] The AIUM Statement on In Vitro Biological Effects
(see Table 7.10) describes limitations in the applicability of in vitro experiments to the clinical environment.

Many studies have been conducted using many endpoints in experi-
mental animals, mostly mice and rats. These data are summarized by the
AIUM Statement on In Vivo Mammalian Bioeffects (see Table 7.7).[62−64,71]
The AIUM statement yields values of 0.1 and 1.0 W/cm^2 SPTA intensity

for unfocused and focused beams, respectively, below which no independently confirmed significant biologic effects in mammalian tissues have been observed. Figure 7.34[67] illustrates the intensity levels described in the AIUM statement. In addition, the minimum levels required for focal lesions[63] are shown on the figure for comparison.

SPTA intensity is used in the AIUM Statement on Mammalian Bioeffects and relates well to a thermal mechanism of interaction. It is the output intensity most commonly presented. Table 7.11 gives a compilation of ranges of SPTA intensities.[72-83] It can be seen that output intensities have a wide range, with the highest being 250,000 times the lowest. Imaging instruments dominate the lower portion of the range while doppler instruments dominate the higher portion.

These output intensity measurements are usually made with the use of hydrophones (see Section 7.2) and radiation force balances located in the beam in a water path. Attenuation in water is low compared to that in tissues so that an intensity at a comparable location within tissue would

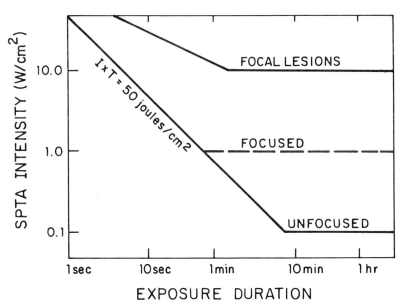

EXPOSURE DURATION

Figure 7.34. Comparison of the minimum SPTA intensities required for ultrasonic bioeffects specified in AIUM Statement on Mammalian Bioeffects. The minimum levels required for focal lesions[63] are also shown on the figure for comparison. Note that logarithmic scaling has been used for the axes of this figure so that the horizontal lines are separated by factors of ten in intensity. (From AIUM: Bioeffects considerations for the safety of diagnostic ultrasound. J Ultrasound Med 7(9): Supplement, 1988. Reprinted with permission.)

Table 7.11
Compilation of Instrument Output
SPTA Intensity (mW/cm^2) Ranges*

All instruments	0.01–2500
Imaging instruments	0.01–680
Scanning	0.01–440
Linear array	0.01–48
Phased array	0.1–85
Mechanical	0.1–440
Stopped	0.5–680
Linear array	3.8–332
Phased array	10.1–240
Mechanical	1.6–680
Static	0.5–200
Doppler instruments	0.6–2500
CW obstetrics	0.6–80
CW cardiac/PV	20.0–2500
Pulsed	40.0–1945

*From References 72–83.

be less than that in water. Models for accounting for the tissue attenuation have been proposed.[84,85] These approaches have yielded the following somewhat conflicting conclusions: (1) Total attenuation to the human fetus averages approximately 11 dB at 3.5 MHz. (2) A realistic estimate of the minimum expected attenuation in early pregnancy is, in dB, one or two times the frequency in MHz.

To compare instrument output intensities with mechanistic predictions and observations (see Tables 7.4 and 7.5) and with experimental bioeffects (see Table 7.7), let us assume a frequency of 3.5 MHz and a 7 dB attenuation. This corresponds to an intensity reduction of 80 percent. Reducing the values in Table 7.11 by 80 percent yields upper limits as given in Table 7.12. Because most of the bioeffects studies were done in small animals, such as mice and rats, the attenuation would be negligible and the values in Table 7.12 can be compared to the AIUM statement value of 1 W/cm^2 (see Table 7.7) for focused beams since virtually all diagnostic ultrasound uses focused beams. It can be seen from this comparison that on the basis of experimental animal studies, clinical bioeffects would not be expected to occur from outputs of current and past diagnostic instrumentation. Note that doppler instruments do yield the highest reported intensities. At a recent symposium on Safety and Standardization in Medical Ultrasound sponsored by the World Federation for Ultrasound in Medicine and Biology, pulsed doppler SPTA intensities higher than 2 W/cm^2 were reported.[86]

Table 7.12
Upper Limits of SPTA Intensity (mW/cm^2) in Table 7.11 Decreased by 7 dB to Account for Human Tissue Attenuation*

All instruments	500
Imaging instruments	136
Scanning	88
Stopped	136
Doppler instruments	500
CW	500
Pulsed	389

*From References 72–83.

7.4
Safety

For consideration of the safety of diagnostic ultrasound, an attempt must be made to relate knowledge of bioeffects to the clinical situation (Fig. 7.35). There are three questions that arise when an attempt is made to accomplish this:

1. Do any of the bioeffects that have occurred under experimental conditions constitute a hazard to a human in the clinical setting?
2. Are the acoustic parameters at the site of the bioeffect in experimental animals comparable to those at the appropriate site of concern in the human body during diagnosis?
3. Do the continuous-wave conditions of most experimental studies provide any useful information for the pulsed ultrasound of clinical diagnosis?

These questions remain largely unanswered. As there is no satisfying response to question 1, an attempt must be made to determine if *any* bioeffects observed in experimental animals are likely to occur clinically. This brings us to the difficulties of questions 2 and 3. The response to question 2 is that in human applications of ultrasound, the organs of concern are

Figure 7.35. Relating bioeffects information to risk determination. Unanswered questions limit our ability to determine the relationship thoroughly.

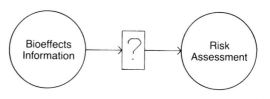

normally farther from the sound source (a longer attenuating sound path is involved). Also, a smaller organ volume fraction is exposed because the organs are larger than those of the experimental animals. These considerations may provide some (unknown) safety factors for the diagnostic situation. Concerning question 3, it is not known whether or not short diagnostic pulses of low duty factor can produce bioeffects under clinical conditions and whether or not repair could occur between pulses.

Several studies of an epidemiologic nature have been conducted and published.[63,64,71] These have been reviewed by Ziskin and Petitti,[87] who concluded that "epidemiologic studies and surveys and widespread clinical usage over 25 years have yielded no evidence of any adverse effect from diagnostic ultrasound." The most recent of these studies is that of Lyons.[88] He and his colleagues studied the head circumference, height, and weight of 149 sibling pairs of the same sex, one of whom had been exposed to diagnostic ultrasound in utero. No statistically significant differences of head circumference at birth or of height and weight between birth and 6 years of age were found between ultrasound exposed and unexposed siblings. Although these studies have limitations and some flaws, they have not indicated risk in the clinical use of diagnostic ultrasound (see Table 7.6). Such risk, if it does exist, may have eluded detection up to this point because it is either subtle, delayed, or of an incidence rate close to normal values. As more sensitive endpoints are studied over longer periods of time or with larger populations, such risk(s) may be identified. On the other hand, studies may not yield any positive effects, thus strengthening the possibility that diagnostic ultrasound is without risk. In the meantime, with no known risk and known benefit to the procedure, a conservative approach to doppler ultrasound should be used.[65,68-71,83,89,90] That is, doppler should be used when medically indicated with minimum exposure of the patient and fetus. Exposure is minimized by minimizing instrument output intensity and by minimizing exposure time during a study. Doppler instrument outputs can be significantly higher than those for imaging (see Table 7.11). It seems most likely that the greatest potential for risk in ultrasound diagnosis (although no specific risk has been identified even in this case) is for fetal or neonatal doppler studies. These combine potentially high output intensities with stationary geometry and the (presumably more sensitive) fetus or neonatal brain. It should be emphasized that color-flow imaging uses a scanning beam just as sonography does so that the potential risk situation in this case appears to be less serious than for conventional doppler spectral analysis.

Tables 7.8 and 7.9 present AIUM statements relevant to the clinical use of diagnostic ultrasound. Extensive mechanistic, in vitro, in vivo, and epidemiologic studies have revealed no known risk with current ultrasound instrumentation used in medical diagnosis, both imaging and flow-

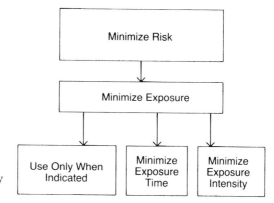

Figure 7.36. Minimize risk by minimizing exposure.

metry. However, a prudent and conservative approach to ultrasound safety is to assume that there may be unidentified risks that should be minimized in medically indicated ultrasound studies by minimizing exposure time and intensity. In short, we should minimize (unknown, but potentially nonzero) risk by minimizing exposure (Fig. 7.36).

7.5
Review

Artifacts with doppler ultrasound include aliasing, range ambiguity, image and doppler signal mirroring, spectral trace mirroring, and 60-Hz interference. Aliasing is the most common artifact. It occurs when the doppler shift frequency exceeds half the pulse repetition frequency. It can be reduced or eliminated by increasing the pulse repetition frequency or doppler angle, using baseline shift, reducing operating frequency, or using a continuous-wave instrument.

Doppler phantoms of two types are available: those that use a blood-mimicking fluid and those that use a moving string. Imaging phantoms and test objects provide checks of axial and lateral resolution, range and registration accuracy, dead zone, compensation, sensitivity, and dynamic range of duplex instruments. Hydrophones are used to measure the acoustic output of diagnostic instruments.

No independently confirmed significant bioeffects in mammalian tissues exposed to focused beams of SPTA intensity below 1 W/cm^2 have occurred. This indicates that with some doppler instruments that operate at higher intensities (as much as 2 W/cm^2), it may be possible to produce some bioeffects in small animals. There is, however, no evidence that they occur in humans. Several epidemiologic studies have indicated no risk with the use of diagnostic ultrasound. Because there is limited specific knowledge, the conservative approach is taken: Use diagnostic ultrasound with minimum exposure when medical benefit is expected from the procedure.

Exercises

7.1 The most common artifact encountered in doppler ultrasound is
  a. aliasing
  b. range ambiguity
  c. spectrum mirror image
  d. location mirror image
  e. electromagnetic interference

7.2 Which of the following can reduce or eliminate aliasing?
  a. increase pulse repetition frequency
  b. increase doppler angle
  c. increase operating frequency
  d. use continuous wave
  e. more than one of the above

7.3 Which of the following can decrease or eliminate aliasing?
  a. decrease pulse repetition frequency
  b. decrease doppler angle
  c. increase operating frequency
  d. baseline shifting
  e. more than one of the above

7.4 To avoid aliasing, a signal voltage must be sampled at least _____ times per cycle.
  a. 1
  b. 2
  c. 3
  d. 4
  e. 5

7.5 If the highest doppler shift frequency present in a signal exceeds _____ the pulse repetition frequency, aliasing will occur.
  a. one tenth
  b. one half
  c. 2 times
  d. 5 times
  e. 10 times

7.6 When a pulse is emitted before all the echoes from the previous pulse have been received, which artifact occurs?

    a. aliasing
    b. range ambiguity
    c. spectrum mirror image
    d. location mirror image
    e. speckle

7.7 When receiver gain is set too high, which artifact is likely to occur?
    a. aliasing
    b. range ambiguity
    c. spectrum mirror image
    d. location mirror image
    e. speckle

7.8 When a strong reflector is located in the scan plane, which of the following artifacts is likely to occur?
    a. aliasing
    b. range ambiguity
    c. spectrum mirror image
    d. location mirror image
    e. speckle

7.9 Constructive and destructive interference of simultaneously arriving echoes produces which artifact?
    a. aliasing
    b. range ambiguity
    c. spectrum mirror image
    d. location mirror image
    e. speckle

7.10 Which of the following decreases the likelihood of range ambiguity artifact?
    a. decreasing operating frequency
    b. decreasing pulse repetition frequency
    c. decreasing doppler angle
    d. baseline shift
    e. increasing pulser output

7.11 Range ambiguity can occur in which of the following?
    a. imaging instruments
    b. duplex instruments
    c. pulsed-doppler instruments
    d. color-flow instruments
    e. all of the above

7.12 Range ambiguity produces which error in echo presentation?
    a. range too long
    b. range too short
    c. intensity too high

d. doppler shift too high

e. doppler shift too low

7.13 If a pulse is emitted 65 microseconds after the previous one, echoes returning from beyond _____ cm will produce range ambiguity.

    a. 1

    b. 2

    c. 3

    d. 4

    e. 5

7.14 To avoid aliasing and range ambiguity, if the maximum depth is 5 cm, frequency is 2 MHz, and doppler angle is zero, what is the maximum flow speed?

    a. 100 cm/s

    b. 200 cm/s

    c. 300 cm/s

    d. 400 cm/s —

    e. 500 cm/s

7.15 Does solving aliasing by decreasing operating frequency increase the possibility of range ambiguity artifact?

7.16 If operating frequency is increased to decrease the possibility of range ambiguity (by increasing attenuation), does the possibility of aliasing increase?

7.17 If a pulsed doppler sample volume is located at a depth of 8 cm, the sampled echoes arrive at what time following the emission of the pulse?

    a. 25 μs

    b. 50 μs

    c. 75 μs

    d. 104 μs

    e. 117 μs

7.18 In Exercise 7.17, if the pulse repetition frequency is set at 11 kHz, a second gate would be located at what depth?

    a. 1 cm

    b. 2 cm

    c. 3 cm

    d. 4 cm

    e. 5 cm

7.19 If the pulse repetition frequency is 4 kHz, which of the following doppler shifts will alias?

    a. 1 kHz

    b. 2 kHz

    c. 3 kHz

d. 4 kHz

e. more than one of the above

7.20 If the pulse repetition frequency is 10 kHz, which of the following doppler shifts will alias?

    a. 1 kHz

    b. 2 kHz

    c. 3 kHz

    d. 4 kHz

    e. none of the above

7.21 Connect the dots (samples) in Figure 7.37 to get the doppler shift frequency. How many cycles are in each example?

    a. _____

    b. _____

    c. _____

    d. _____

    e. _____

7.22 The frequencies that were sampled in Exercise 7.21 are shown in Figure 7.38. In which example(s) has aliasing occurred?

7.23 Doppler flow phantoms fall into two groups: those that use a blood-mimicking _____ and those that use a moving _____ for scattering the ultrasound.

7.24 The 100-mm test object contains several stainless steel _____ immersed in a mixture of algae inhibitor,

Figure 7.37. Illustrations for Exercise 7.21.

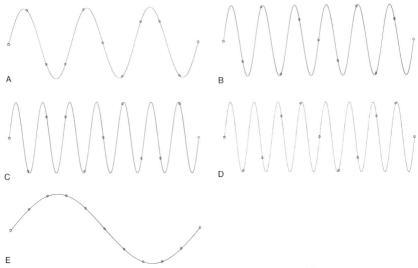

Figure 7.38. Illustrations for Exercise 7.22.

_____, and _____ that has a propagation speed of 1.54 mm/μs.

7.25 Match the parameters measured with the rod groups used (see Fig. 7.12). (Answers may be used more than once.)

_____ **a.** axial resolution   **1.** rod group (a)
_____ **b.** lateral resolution   **2.** rod group (b)
_____ **c.** range accuracy   **3.** rod group (c)
_____ **d.** registration accuracy   **4.** rod group (d)
_____ **e.** dead zone   **5.** rod group (e)
_____ **f.** compensation   **6.** all rods
_____ **g.** sensitivity   **7.** any rods
_____ **h.** dynamic range

7.26 Match the parameters measured with the types of observation modes. (Answers may be used more than once.)

_____ **a.** axial resolution   **1.** gain or attenuator settings
_____ **b.** lateral resolution   **2.** first rod imaged
_____ **c.** range accuracy   **3.** rod distances from transducer
_____ **d.** dead zone   in the display
_____ **e.** compensation   **4.** minimum spacing of
_____ **f.** sensitivity   separately displayed rods
_____ **g.** dynamic range

7.27 Test objects are available commercially. True or false?

7.28 Results using a test object are relatively insensitive to temperature. True or false?

7.29 The speed of sound in the recommended alcohol and water mixture of the AIUM test object varies by less than _____ percent when the temperature is changed by 5°C.

7.30 A limitation to the use of rod group (b) for lateral resolution measurement is that it yields an observtion at only one _____ from the transducer.

7.31 To solve the difficulty in Exercise 7.30, rod group (c) may be used to yield beam width information at several _____.

7.32 Tissue-equivalent phantoms attempt to represent some acoustic property of _____.

7.33 The AIUM test object is an example of a tissue-equivalent phantom. True or false?

7.34 Which of these devices measure(s) parameters related to beam profiling?
   a. 100-mm test object
   b. SUAR test object
   c. hydrophone
   d. both a and c
   e. both b and c

7.35 Reflection profilers plot acoustic amplitude or intensity across the beam at several distances from the transducer. True or false?

7.36 The following are often supplied with beam profiles to show their characteristics:
   a. pulsers
   b. transducers
   c. receivers
   d. displays
   e. both a and c

7.37 A spectrum analyzer is used to determine _____.
   a. color spectrum
   b. impedance spectrum
   c. lateral resolution
   d. frequency spectrum
   e. all of the above

7.38 Using a hydrophone, which of the following can be measured or calculated? (More than one correct answer.)
   a. impedance
   b. amplitude
   c. frequency
   d. duty factor
   e. pulse repetition frequency

7.39 Hydrophones are available commercially and are relatively simple to use. True or false?

7.40 A hydrophone contains a small _____ element.

7.41 Because of its small size, a hydrophone can measure spatial details of a sound beam. True or false?

7.42 A hydrophone
  a. interacts with light
  b. produces a voltage
  c. measures intensity directly
  d. measures total energy
  e. none of the above

7.43 Heating depends most directly on
  a. SATA intensity
  b. SATP intensity
  c. SPTP intensity

7.44 When SPTA intensities of pulsed and continuous-wave ultrasound are compared, the appropriate time to be used is
  a. the total exposure time
  b. the sound-on time

7.45 When SPTP intensity of pulsed ultrasound is compared with SPTA intensity of continuous-wave ultrasound, the appropriate time to be used is
  a. the total exposure time
  b. the sound-on time

7.46 The sound-on time is the total time multipled by
  a. beam uniformity ratio
  b. pulse repetition frequency
  c. doppler shift
  d. reflection coefficient
  e. duty factor

7.47 The available epidemiologic data are sufficient to make a final judgment on the safety of diagnostic ultrasound. True or false?

7.48 Exposure is minimized by using diagnostic ultrasound
  a. only when indicated
  b. with minimum intensity
  c. with minimum time
  d. all of the above
  e. none of the above

7.49 Match these devices or phenomena with what they measure. (Answers may be used more than once.)

_____ **a.** beam profiler	**1.** diagnostic instrument imaging performance
_____, _____ **b.** 100-mm test object	**2.** transducer beam characteristics
_____, _____ **c.** hydrophone	**3.** diagnostic instrument acoustic output

7.50 Match the following with the components about which they usually provide information:

_____ a. hydrophone

_____ b. beam profiler

_____ c. 100-mm test object

1. diagnostic instrument as whole
2. pulser and transducer
3. transducer
4. transducer and receiver
5. receiver and display

7.51 There is no possible hazard involved in the diagnostic use of ultrasound. True or false?

7.52 Ultrasound should not be used as a diagnostic tool because of the bioeffects it can produce. True or false?

7.53 No independently confirmed significant bioeffects in mammalian tissues have been reported at intensities below

a. 10 W/cm^2 SPTP

b. 100 mW/cm^2 SPTA

c. 10 mW/cm^2 SPTA

d. 10 mW/cm^2 SATA

e. 1 mW/cm^2 SATP

7.54 Is there any knowledge of what types of injuries or risks occur with diagnostic ultrasound in patients and under what conditions? Yes or no?

7.55 Is there any knowledge of any bioeffects that ultrasound produces in small animals under experimental conditions? Yes or no?

7.56 Which of the following are mechanisms by which ultrasound can produce bioeffects?
(More than one correct answer.)

a. direction ionization

b. absorption

c. photoelectric effect

d. cavitation

e. Compton effect

7.57 Which of the following relates to heating?

a. impedance

b. sound speed

c. absorption

d. refraction

e. diffraction

7.58 The SPTA intensity below which bioeffects in experimental animals have not been confirmed in the 0.5 to 10 MHz frequency range for focused beams is

a. 100 μW/cm^2

b. 1 mW/cm^2

c. 1 W/cm^2

d. 100 W/cm^2

e. 100 kW/cm^2

7.59 The following endpoint is documented in the scientific literature well enough that a risk assessment for diagnostic ultrasound can be based on it:

a. fetal weight

b. sister chromatid exchange

c. fetal abnormalities

d. carcinogenesis

e. none

7.60 More than one epidemiologic study has shown a statistically significant effect of ultrasound exposure on which of the following endpoints?

a. fetal activity

b. birth weight

c. fetal abnormalities

d. dyslexia

e. none

7.61 Which of the following acoustic parameters have been documented in ultrasound epidemiologic studies published thus far?

a. frequency

b. exposure time

c. intensity and pulsing conditions

d. scanning patterns

e. none

7.62 A device commonly used to measure output of diagnostic ultrasound instruments is

a. hydrophone

b. optical interferometer

c. Geiger counter

d. photoelectric cell

e. absorption radiometer

7.63 A typical output intensity (SPTA) for an ultrasound imaging instrument is

a. 1540 W

b. 13 kW/mm^2

c. 3.5 MHz

d. 1 mW/cm^2

e. 2 dB/cm

7.64 Which of the following typically have the highest output intensity?

a. fetal monitor doppler

b. duplex pulsed doppler

c. static imager

d. mechanical real-time imager

e. phased-array, real-time imager

7.65 The attenuation of 3.5 MHz ultrasound in soft tissue is such that the intensity at a depth of 8 cm is approximately what fraction of that at the transducer face (skin surface)?

a. 90 percent

b. 50 percent

c. 20 percent

d. 4 percent

e. 0.01 percent

7.66 As far as we know now, which of the following is the most correct and informative response to a patient's question, "Will this hurt me or my baby?"

a. no

b. yes

c. I don't know

d. the risks are well understood but the benefits always outweigh them

e. there is no known risk with ultrasound imaging as applied currently

7.67 In order to minimize whatever (unidentified) risk there may be with ultrasound imaging, the following should be done. (More than one correct answer.)

a. scan for family album pictures

b. scan to determine fetal sex

c. minimize exposure time

d. scan for medical indication only

e. minimize exposure intensity

7.68 Which of the following controls affect instrument output intensity?

a. dynamic range, compression

b. transmit, output

c. near gain, far gain

d. overall gain

e. slope, TGC

7.69 Which of the following are correct for a duplex-pulsed doppler instrument? (More than one correct answer.)

a. tissue anywhere in the doppler beam is exposed to ultrasound

b. tissue anywhere in the imaging plane is exposed to ultrasound

c. imaging intensities are higher than for conventional real-time instruments

d. doppler intensities are higher than for continuous-wave fetal monitoring

   e. tissue is exposed to the doppler beam only at the location of the gate

7.70 The tissue of greatest concern with regard to bioeffects in an abdominal scan is

   a. spleen

   b. pancreas

   c. liver

   d. kidney

   e. fetus

7.71 Would it be wise to substitute a duplex-pulsed doppler device for an inoperative fetal monitor for long-term (e.g., 24-hour) monitoring in labor and delivery?

   a. yes

   b. no

   c. depends on frame rate of image

   d. depends on frequency of doppler beam

   e. depends on gate location

7.72 Which of the following is (are) likely to be exposed to ultrasound during a diagnostic study?

   a. patient

   b. sonographer

   c. sonologist

   d. observers in the room

   e. more than one of the above

Chapter 8

Summary

By sending short pulses of ultrasound into the body and using reflected and scattered sound received from tissue interfaces and from within tissues to produce images of internal structures, ultrasound is used as a medical diagnostic tool. Ultrasound is a wave of traveling acoustic variables described by frequency, wavelength, propagation speed, amplitude, intensity, and attenuation.

Pulsed ultrasound is used in sonography. It is described, additionally, by pulse repetition frequency and spatial pulse length. Diagnostic ultrasound commonly uses frequencies from 2 to 10 MHz.

For perpendicular incidence at boundaries, reflections are produced if media impedances are different. For oblique incidence, refraction occurs if media propagation speeds are different. Scattering occurs at rough boundaries and within heterogeneous media. The distance to reflectors is determined by round-trip travel time.

Transducers convert electric energy to ultrasound energy and vice versa by piezoelectricity. Axial resolution is equal to one half the pulse length, which can be reduced by damping and increasing frequency (improving resolution). Lateral resolution is equal to beam diameter, which can be reduced (improving resolution) by focusing. Disc transducers produce sound beams with near and far zones. Focusing can only be

195

accomplished in the near zone of the comparable unfocused transducer. Arrays can scan, steer, and shape beams repeatedly, permitting dynamic imaging. Dynamic imaging can also be accomplished with mechanically driven single-element transducers or mirrors.

Pulse-echo systems use the amplitude, direction, and arrival time of echoes to produce images. Imaging systems consist of pulser, transducer, receiver, memory, and display. The pulser delivers the energizing voltages to the transducer that responds by producing ultrasound pulses. Receivers amplify voltages representing returning echoes and compensate for attenuation. Digital memories store gray-scale image information and permit display on a television monitor. The number of bits per pixel in the digital memory determines the number of gray shades that can be displayed by the system. Dynamic imaging instruments display a rapid sequence of static pictures (frames).

Display artifacts include reverberation, refraction, mirror image, shadowing, and enhancement. The latter two are useful in evaluation of masses producing them.

Fluids are substances that flow. Blood is a liquid that flows through the vascular system under the influence of pulsatile pressure as provided by the beating heart. Volume flow rate is proportional to pressure difference at the ends of a tube and inversely proportional to the flow resistance. The flow resistance increases with tube length and decreases (strongly) with tube diameter. Flow resistance is proportional to fluid viscosity. Five flow classifications include plug, laminar (parabolic), steady, disturbed, and turbulent. In a stenosis, flow speeds up, pressure drops, and the flow is disturbed. If flow speed exceeds a critical value as described by the reynolds number, the onset of turbulence occurs. Pulsatile flow is common in arterial circulation. It results in added diastolic flow and flow reversal depending on location within the arterial system. The fluid inertia and vessel compliance are characteristics that are important in determining flow with pulsatile driving pressure.

The doppler effect is a change in frequency or wavelength resulting from motion. In medical ultrasound applications, the motion is either that of the heart or blood flow in circulation. The change in frequency of the returning echoes with respect to the emitted frequency is called the doppler shift. For flow toward the transducer it is positive; for flow away it is negative. The doppler shift depends upon the speed of the scatterers of sound, the angle between their direction and that of the sound propagation, and the operating frequency of the doppler system. Thus, reporting a doppler shift frequency without specifying the operating frequency and doppler angle is incomplete. A moving scatterer of sound produces a double doppler shift. Greater flow speeds and smaller doppler angles produce larger doppler shifts but not stronger echoes. Higher operating frequencies produce larger doppler shifts. Typical ranges of flow speeds (10 to 100 cm/s), doppler angle (30 to 60 degrees), and operating frequencies (2 to 10 MHz) yield doppler shifts in the range of 100 Hz to 11 kHz for vascular studies. In doppler echocardiography where zero angle and speeds of a few meters per second can be encountered, doppler shifts can be as high as 30 kHz.

Doppler instruments make use of the doppler shift to yield information regarding motion and flow. Continuous-wave systems provide motion and flow information without depth information or selection capability. Pulsed-doppler systems provide depth information and the ability to select depth from which doppler information is received. Spectral analysis provides visual information on the distribution of received doppler-shift frequencies resulting from the distribution of scatterer speeds and directions encountered. In addition to audible output, imaging of vessel flow spectra is possible in doppler systems. Combined systems utilizing dynamic sonography and continuous-wave and pulsed-wave doppler are available commercially. Color-flow systems provide displays of two-dimensional, real-time flow superimposed on gray-scale anatomic scans. Flow direction is indicated by the color assignment to the doppler-shifted echoes on the display.

The doppler spectrum is generated by the range of scatterer velocities encountered by the ultrasound beam. It is derived electronically using the fast fourier transform and presented on the display in two forms—power versus doppler shift or doppler shift versus time with brightness indicating power. The latter presentation is, by far, the most commonly used. Flow conditions at the site of measurement are indicated by the width of the spectrum with spectral broadening and loss of window indicative of disturbed and turbulent flow. Flow conditions downstream, particularly distal flow impedance, are indicated by the relationship between peak systolic and end diastolic flow speeds. Various indices for quantitatively presenting this information have been developed. Color-flow instruments do not present spectral information in detail but can indicate regions of spectral broadening with a color tag. Oversimplistic interpretation of spectral traces and color-flow images should be avoided.

Artifacts with doppler ultrasound include aliasing, range ambiguity, image and doppler signal mirroring, spectral trace mirroring, and 60 Hz interference. Aliasing is the most common artifact. It occurs when the doppler shift frequency exceeds half the pulse repetition frequency. It can be reduced or eliminated by increasing the pulse repetition frequency or doppler angle, using baseline shift, reducing operating frequency, or using a continuous-wave instrument.

Doppler phantoms of two types are available: those that use a blood-mimicking fluid and those that use a moving string. Imaging phantoms and test objects provide checks of axial and lateral resolution, range and registration accuracy, dead zone, compensation, sensitivity, and dynamic range of duplex instruments. Hydrophones are used to measure the acoustic output of diagnostic instruments.

No independently confirmed significant bioeffects in mammalian tissues exposed to focused beams of SPTA intensity below 1 W/cm^2 have occurred. This indicates that with some doppler instruments that operate at higher intensities (as much as 2 W/cm^2), it may be possible to produce some bioeffects in small animals. There is, however, no evidence that they occur in humans. Several epidemiologic studies have indicated no risk with the use of diagnostic ultrasound. Because there is limited specific knowledge, the conservative approach is taken: Use diagnostic ultrasound with minimum exposure when benefit is expected from the procedure.

Exercises

8.1 Doppler systems convert _____ _____ information to audible sound or visual display.

8.2 A pulser similar to that used in imaging systems is used in doppler systems. True or false?

8.3 Doppler system transducers may have _____ or _____ elements.

8.4 The receiver in a doppler system compares the _____ of the voltage generator and the voltage from the receiving transducer.

8.5 The doppler shift usually is not in the audible frequency range and must be converted by the receiver to a frequency that can be heard. True or false?

8.6 Doppler shift is determined by reflector _____ and by the cosine of an angle.

8.7 A component that pulsed doppler systems have but continuous-wave doppler systems do not have is the _____.

8.8 A doppler system may have as an output a visual _____.

8.9 In a pulsed doppler system, the pulse repetition frequency is determined by the generator _____, and the source ultrasound frequency is determined by the _____.

8.10 Pulsed doppler systems can give motion information as a function of _____.

8.11 A typical SPTA output intensity for a doppler instrument is 50 mW/cm^2. True or false?

8.12 The sound received by the transducer in a doppler instrument is in the audible frequency range. True or false?

8.13 Frequencies used in doppler ultrasound are in approximately the same range as those for pulse echo imaging. True or false?

8.14 If the incident frequency is 4 MHz, the reflector speed is 100 cm/s, and the angle between beam and motion directions is 60 degrees, the doppler shift is _____ kHz.

8.15 There is no problem in Exercise 8.14 with aliasing with a pulse frequency of 10 kHz. True or false?

8.16 If there were a problem in Exercise 8.15, _____
_____ doppler ultrasound could be used to avoid it.

8.17 Color-flow instruments use
    a. continuous-wave doppler
    b. pulsed doppler
    c. compressed doppler
    d. all of the above
    e. none of the above

8.18 Increasing the frequency
    a. improves the resolution
    b. increases the half-intensity depth
    c. increases refraction
    d. both a and b
    e. both a and c

8.19 Increasing the pulse repetition frequency
    a. improves resolution
    b. increases maximum unambiguous depth
    c. decreases maximum unambiguous depth
    d. both a and b
    e. both a and c

8.20 Increasing the intensity produced by the transducer
    a. is accomplished by increasing the pulser voltage
    b. increases the sensitivity of the system
    c. increases the probability of bioeffects
    d. all of the above
    e. none of the above

8.21 Increasing the spatial pulse length
    a. is accomplished by transducer damping
    b. is accompanied by decreased pulse duration
    c. improves the axial resolution
    d. all of the above
    e. none of the above

8.22 Dynamic imaging is made possible by
    a. scan converters
    b. mechanically driven transducers
    c. gray-scale display
    d. arrays
    e. both b and d

8.23 The 100-mm test object measures
  a. resolution
  b. pulse duration
  c. SATA intensity
  d. wavelength
  e. all of the above

8.24 The following measure(s) acoustic output:
  a. hydrophone
  b. scan converter
  c. 100-mm test object
  d. all of the above
  e. none of the above

8.25 Ultrasound bioeffects
  a. do not occur
  b. do not occur with diagnostic instruments
  c. are not confirmed below 100 mW/cm^2 SPTA
  d. both b and c
  e. none of the above

8.26 The diagnostic ultrasound frequency range is
  a. 2 to 10 mHz
  b. 2 to 10 kHz
  c. 2 to 10 mHz
  d. 3 to 15 kHz
  e. none of the above

8.27 Small transducers always produce smaller beam diameters. True or false?

8.28 No reflection occurs if media impedances are equal. True or false?

8.29 No refraction occurs if media impedances are equal. True or false?

8.30 Gray-scale display is made possible by
  a. array transducers
  b. cathode-ray storage tubes
  c. scan converters
  d. both b and c
  e. all of the above

8.31 Attenuation is corrected for by
  a. demodulation
  b. desegregation
  c. decompression
  d. compensation

8.32 The doppler effect for a scatterer moving toward the transducer causes scattered sound (compared with the incident sound) received by the transducer to have _____.
  a. increased intensity
  b. decreased intensity

    c. increased impedance
    d. increased frequency
    e. decreased impedance

8.33 An ultrasound instrument that could represent 64 shades of gray would require an eight-bit memory. True or false?

8.34 Continuous-wave sound is used in _____.
    a. all imaging instruments
    b. some imaging instruments
    c. all doppler instruments
    d. some doppler instruments
    e. none of the above

8.35 An advantage of continuous-wave doppler instruments is that they have _____.
    a. no aliasing
    b. depth information and selectivity
    c. bidirectional information
    d. amplitude information
    e. all of the above

8.36 An advantage of pulsed doppler instruments is that they have _____.
    a. no aliasing
    b. depth information
    c. bidirectional information
    d. amplitude information
    e. all of the above

8.37 A digital memory with one bit per pixel would have a _____ display.
    a. bidirectional
    b. biscattering
    c. bistable

8.38 If a transducer element 19 mm in diameter is focused to produce a minimum beam diameter of 2 mm, the intensity at the focus is approximately _____ times the intensity at the transducer.
    a. 2
    b. 3
    c. 19
    d. 100
    e. 500

8.39 The largest number that can be stored in a pixel of a seven-bit digital memory is _____.
    a. 16
    b. 32
    c. 127

  d. 255
  e. 256

8.40 Digital calipers provide a measurement of distance between _____.

  a. potentiometers
  b. bits
  c. optical encoders
  d. pixels
  e. all of the above

8.41 Which of the following produce(s) a sector-scan format?

  a. rotating mechanical real-time transducer
  b. oscillating mechanical real-time transducer
  c. phased array
  d. oscillating mirror
  e. all of the above

8.42 A digital imaging instrument divides the cross-sectional image into _____.

  a. frequencies
  b. bits
  c. pixels
  d. binaries
  e. wavelengths

8.43 If the thickness of a transducer element is decreased, the frequency is _____.

  a. increased
  b. unchanged
  c. decreased
  d. intensified
  e. none of the above

8.44 In Exercise 8.43 the near-zone length is _____.

  a. increased
  b. unchanged
  c. decreased
  d. intensified
  e. none of the above

8.45 With increased damping, which of the following is increased?

  a. bandwidth
  b. pulse duration
  c. spatial pulse length
  d. Q factor
  e. all of the above

8.46 As frequency is increased, which of the following is (are) decreased?

  a. propagation speed
  b. half-intensity depth

    c. imaging depth

    d. more than one of the above

    e. none of the above

8.47 A five-bit memory can store which of the following numbers?

    a. 64

    b. 32

    c. 31

    d. 55

    e. all of the above

8.48 Television monitors produce _____ frames per second.

    a. 10

    b. 24

    c. 30

    d. 60

    e. none of the above

8.49 Duplex doppler instruments include _____.

    a. pulsed doppler

    b. continuous-wave doppler

    c. static imaging

    d. dynamic imaging

    e. more than one of the above

8.50 If the doppler shifts from normal and from stenotic carotid arteries are 4 kHz and 10 kHz, respectively, for which will there be a problem with a pulse repetition frequency of 7 kHz?

    a. normal

    b. stenotic

    c. both

    d. neither

8.51 Compensation (swept gain) makes up for the fact that reflections from deeper reflectors arrive at the transducer later. True or false?

8.52 Which of the following affects contrast resolution?

    a. number of pixels

    b. number of bits per pixel

    c. pulse duration

    d. frequency

    e. focusing

8.53 Which of the following requires a phased array as a receiving transducer?

    a. dynamic range

    b. dynamic imaging

    c. dynamic focusing

    d. none of the above

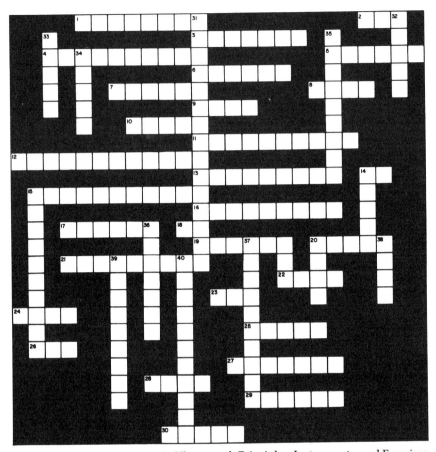

(From Kremkau FW: Diagnostic Ultrasound: Principles, Instruments, and Exercises, 3rd Edition. Philadelphia, WB Saunders, 1989)

8.54 Across:
1. Referring to sound
2. Abbreviation for cosine
3. Not perpendicular to a boundary
4. Occurs at boundaries with perpendicular incidence
5. Material through which sound is passing
6. Pulsed doppler requires _____ the receiver.
7. The duty _____ is sound-on fraction.
8. Beam diameter decreases in the _____ zone.
9. Intensity is power divided by _____.

10. Reflector motion produces a doppler _____.
11. Sound of frequency 20 kHz and higher
12. Parallel to sound direction
13. Maximum variation of an acoustic variable
14. Abbreviation for continuous wave
15. Attenuation _____ is given in decibels per centimeter.
16. Power divided by area
17. Reciprocal of frequency
18. The range equation gives distance _____ a reflector.
19. Perpendicular to a boundary
20. Displacement divided by time
21. Propagation speed depends on density and _____.
22. _____ scale displays several values of spot brightness.
23. Beam diameter increases in the _____ zone.
24. Force times displacement
25. Axial resolution depends on spatial _____ length.
26. Abbreviation for sine
27. Reflected frequency minus incident frequency equals _____ shift.
28. A traveling variation
29. Capability for doing work
30. Complete variation of a wave variable

Down:
14. One hertz is one _____ per second.
15. The abbreviation cw stands for _____ wave.
20. A line produced on a display is called a _____ line.
31. (A message for you)
32. Traveling wave of acoustic variables
33. Transducer assembly containing more than one element
34. _____ length is the distance from a focused transducer to minimum beam diameter.
35. Density times propagation speed
36. Mass divided by volume
37. Another name for a hydrophone
38. Pulse duration divided by pulse repetition period is _____ factor.
39. Reciprocal of period
40. Ability of an imaging system to detect weak reflections

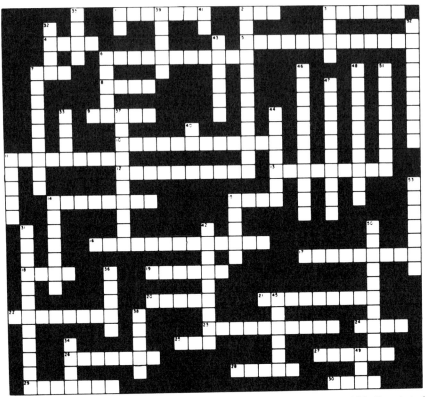

(From Kremkau FW: Crossword puzzle. Med Ultrasound 4:38, 1980. Reprinted with permission of John Wiley & Sons, Inc.)

8.55 Across:
1. Ratio of largest to smallest power that a system can handle is called _____ range.
2. At a distance of one near-zone length from a disc transducer, beam diameter is approximately equal to disc diameter divided by _____.

3. Passing only reflections that arrive at a certain time after the transducer has produced a pulse is called _____.
4. Continuously displaying moving structures is called _____ time imaging.
5. Increasing small voltages to larger ones.
6. The speed with which a wave moves through a medium is called _____ speed.
7. The region of a sound beam where beam diameter increases with distance from the transducer is called the _____ zone.
8. Another word for a reflection
9. Acoustic means having to do with _____.
10. If propagation speeds of two media are equal, incidence angle equals _____ angle.
11. A device that stores a gray-scale image and allows it to be displayed on a television monitor is called a scan _____.
12. Conversion of sound to heat
13. Power divided by area
14. An echo-free region on a display is called _____.
15. The fraction of time that pulsed ultrasound is actually on is called _____ factor.
16. The AIUM statement on bioeffects says that there have been no _____ confirmed significant bioeffects below 100 mW/cm^2.
17. Density multiplied by sound propagation speed
18. Displaying several values of spot brightness is called a _____ scale.
19. If no reflection occurs at a boundary, this always means that media impedances are equal in the case of _____ incidence.
20. A few cycles of ultrasound may be called an ultrasound _____.
21. Maximum variation of an acoustic variable or voltage
22. Reverberations are also called _____ reflections.
23. A device that converts energy from one form to another
24. Prefix meaning 1000
25. Abbreviation for megahertz
26. _____ incidence is when the sound direction is not perpendicular to the boundary of the medium.
27. Capability of doing work
28. Number of complete scans displayed per unit time in a real-time system is called the _____ rate.
29. Perpendicular to the direction of sound travel
30. A unit for impedance

Down:

1. Abbreviation for decibel
2. Sound _____ through a medium improves as attenuation decreases
3. Ratio of output to input electrical power for an amplifier
6. A Greek prefix meaning pressure
7. Number of cycles per unit time
11. One hertz is one _____ per second.
14. An _____ array is made up of ring-shaped elements.
15. Half-intensity _____ decreases with increasing frequency.
31. Along the direction of sound travel (axial)
32. Focusing produces decreased beam _____.
33. A sound _____ is a traveling variation of acoustic variables.
34. Most two-dimensional imaging is done with B _____ displays.
35. To sweep a sound beam to produce an image
36. Rate at which work is done; rate at which energy is transferred
37. Sound of frequency greater than 20 kHz
38. Concentrate the sound beam into a smaller area
39. A transducer _____ is an assembly containing more than one transducer element.
40. Abbreviation for millimeter
41. Abbreviation for continuous wave
42. Frequency unit
43. A _____ array is made up of rectangular elements in a line.
44. Propagation speed increases with decreasing _____.
45. Material through which a wave travels
46. Decrease of amplitude and intensity as a wave travels through a medium
47. Length of space over which a cycle occurs
48. Change of sound direction on passing from one medium to another
49. A cathode _____ tube is a common display device.
50. Diffusion or redirection of sound in several directions
51. Speed, with direction of motion specified
52. Perpendicular _____ occurs when sound direction is perpendicular to the boundary of the medium.
53. The _____ effect is a frequency change of reflected sound wave due to reflector motion.

8.56 Identify the physical terms, the common measurement units for which are given.

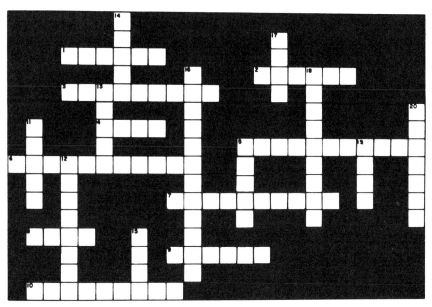

(From Kremkau FW: Ultrapuzzles. Reflections 6:85, 1980. Reprinted with permission of the American Institute of Ultrasound in Medicine)

Across:
1. joule
2. microsecond
3. rayl
4. joule
5. decibel
6. kelvin
7. millimeter
8. gram
9. milliliter
10. hertz

Down:
5. radian
11. meter/second
12. newton/meter^2
13. watt
14. newton
15. decibel
16. meter/second^2
17. centimeter^2
18. watt/centimeter^2
19. second
20. gram/milliliter

8.57 In the following review, blanks need to be filled in. In the figure, begin at the upper left and draw a line to one letter at a time in any direction (horizontal, vertical, or diagonal) to spell out the words for the blanks. All letters are used in a continuous line. Do not cross over your line. Use each letter only once. The words should be found in the same order as they are needed for the blanks.

START

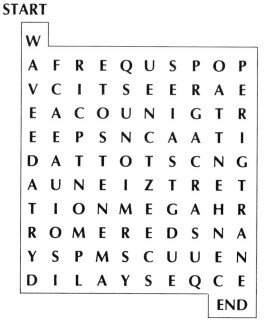

W								
A	F	R	E	Q	U	S	P	O	P
V	C	I	T	S	E	E	R	A	E
E	A	C	O	U	N	I	G	T	R
E	E	P	S	N	C	A	A	T	I
D	A	T	T	O	T	S	C	N	G
A	U	N	E	I	Z	T	R	E	T
T	I	O	N	M	E	G	A	H	R
R	O	M	E	R	E	D	S	N	A
Y	S	P	M	S	C	U	U	E	N
D	I	L	A	Y	S	E	Q	C	E

END

(From Kremkau FW: Diagnostic Ultrasound: Principles, Instruments, and Exercises, 3rd Edition. Philadelphia, WB Saunders, 1989)

Ultrasound is a _____ of traveling _____ variables.

Pulsed ultrasound is commonly used in ultrasound imaging. Pulses contain a range of _____. Soft tissue _____ _____ is 1.54 mm/µs and the _____ coefficient is 0.5 dB/cm for each _____ of frequency. _____ occurs at rough boundaries and within heterogeneous media. _____ convert electric energy to ultrasound energy and vice versa. Imaging systems consist of pulser, transducer, receiver, _____, and _____. Dynamic imaging instruments display a rapid _____ of static pictures.

8.58 Find the following words that are hidden in the puzzle:

aliasing
color-flow
continuous-wave
doppler-angle
doppler-shift
frequency
pulsed-wave
ultrasound

They may appear horizontally, vertically, or diagonally.

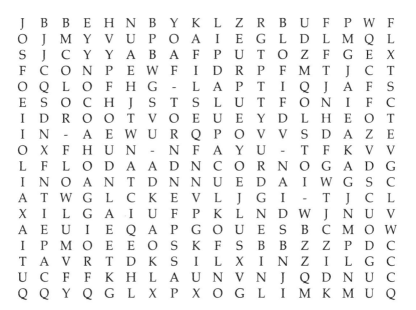

J B B E H N B Y K L Z R B U F P W F
O J M Y V U P O A I E G L D L M Q L
S J C Y Y A B A F P U T O Z F G E X
F C O N P E W F I D R P F M T J C T
O Q L O F H G - L A P T I Q J A F S
E S O C H J S T S L U T F O N I F C
I D R O O T V O E U E Y D L H E O T
I N - A E W U R Q P O V V S D A Z E
O X F H U N - N F A Y U - T F K V V
L F L O D A A D N C O R N O G A D G
I N O A N T D N N U E D A I W G S C
A T W G L C K E V L J G I - T J C L
X I L G A I U F P K L N D W J N U V
A E U I E Q A P G O U E S B C M O W
I P M O E E O S K F S B B Z Z P D C
T A V R T D K S I L X I N Z I L G C
U C F F K H L A U N V N J Q D N U C
Q Q Y Q G L X P X O G L I M K M U Q

8.59 Reflections are produced by changes in
  a. stiffness
  b. density
  c. absorption
  d. attenuation
  e. both a and b
8.60 If no reflection occurs at a boundary, this always means that media impedances are equal in the case of
  a. perpendicular incidence
  b. oblique incidence
  c. refraction
  d. both a and b
  e. both b and c
8.61 If the propagation speeds in two media are equal, the refraction equation states that the incidence angle equals the
  a. reflection angle
  b. transmission angle
  c. doppler angle
  d. both a and b
  e. both b and c
8.62 Velocity is _____.
  a. speed
  b. direction
  c. acceleration

d. a and b

e. all of the above

8.63 Decibels are _____ ratio units.

    a. amplitude

    b. power

    c. neper

    d. more than one of the above

    e. all of the above

8.64 Which of the following can be real-time? (More than one correct answer)

    a. A mode

    b. B mode

    c. B scan

    d. M mode

    e. doppler

8.65 A characteristic of an AIUM 100-mm test object that may produce incorrect results is

    a. weight of the liquid

    b. age of the liquid

    c. sound speed in the liquid

    d. temperature of the rods

    e. none of the above

8.66 The following test(s) can be performed using the AIUM 100-mm test object

    a. dead zone

    b. resolution

    c. registration accuracy

    d. range accuracy

    e. all of the above

8.67 If all six rods of the central groups in an AIUM 100-mm test object appear separately on a display of the object, the axial resolution is

    a. 1 mm

    b. 2 mm

    c. 3 mm

    d. 4 mm

    e. 5 mm

8.68 Which of the following produce(s) a sector scan format?

    a. rotating mechanical real-time transducer

    b. oscillating mechanical real-time transducer

    c. phased array

    d. linear switched array

    e. more than one of the above

8.69 Which of the following produce(s) a rectangular scan format?
    a. rotating mechanical real-time transducer
    b. oscillating mechanical real-time transducer
    c. phased array
    d. linear switched array
    e. more than one of the above

8.70 Gray-scale displays present brightness corresponding to echo
    a. frequency
    b. amplitude
    c. bandwidth
    d. impedance
    e. more than one of the above

8.71 A digital scan converter stores _____ corresponding to echo amplitudes.
    a. numbers
    b. electrical charges
    c. lines
    d. frames
    e. none of the above

8.72 Intensity of returning echoes changes with angle in doppler flow measurements. True or false?

8.73 Intensity of returning echoes changes with flow speed in doppler ultrasound. True or false?

8.74 Figure 8.1 describes which resolution?

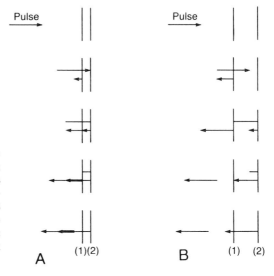

Figure 8.1. Figure for Exercises 8.74 and 8.75. (From Kremkau FW: Basic principles and biological effects of ultrasound. *In* Resnick MI, Sanders RC [eds]: Ultrasound in Urology. Baltimore, Williams & Wilkins, 1979, Reprinted with permission.)

a. axial
b. lateral
c. contrast
d. detail
e. a and d
8.75 In which part of Figure 8.1 (a or b) are the two reflectors resolved?
8.76 In Figure 8.2, give the following:
   a. number of cycles in a pulse
   b. amplitude
   c. wavelength
   d. spatial pulse length
   e. pulse repetition period
   f. pulse repetition frequency
   g. pulse duration

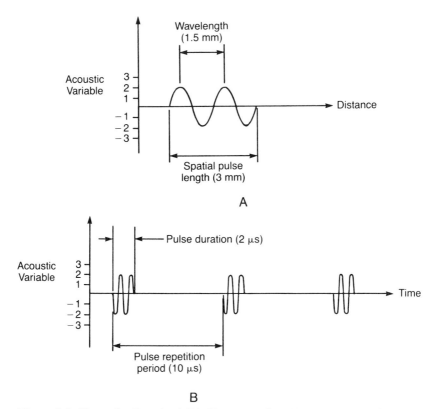

Figure 8.2. Figure for Exercise 8.76. (From Kremkau FW: Basic principles and biological effects of ultrasound. *In* Resnick MI, Sanders RC [eds]: Ultrasound in Urology. Baltimore, Williams & Wilkins, 1979. Reprinted with permission.)

h. period
i. frequency
j. duty factor
k. propagation speed

8.77 In which part of Figure 8.3 (a, b, c) is speed (2) greater than speed (1); is speed (2) less than speed (1); is speed (2) equal to speed (1); is there no refraction?

8.78 Figure 8.4 shows that a higher frequency yields a (longer, shorter) near-zone length and that a larger transducer produces a (longer, shorter) near-zone length. By curving them, which of these transducers (a, b, c, d) can be focused at 25 cm; at 15 cm; at 4 cm?

8.79 In Figure 8.5, the wave type is (continuous-wave, pulsed), if the lower portion of the figure represents 4 ms later than the upper portion, the propagation speed is _____ mm/μs, the wavelength for 1 MHz frequency is _____ mm, and the spatial pulse length is _____ mm.

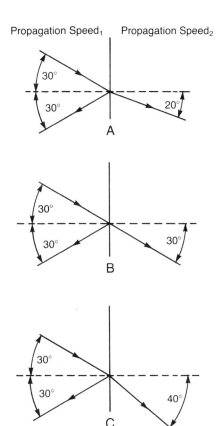

Figure 8.3. Figure for Exercise 8.77. (From Kremkau FW: Basic principles and biological effects of ultrasound. *In* Resnick MI, Sanders RC [eds]: Ultrasound in Urology. Baltimore, Williams & Wilkins, 1979. Reprinted with permission.)

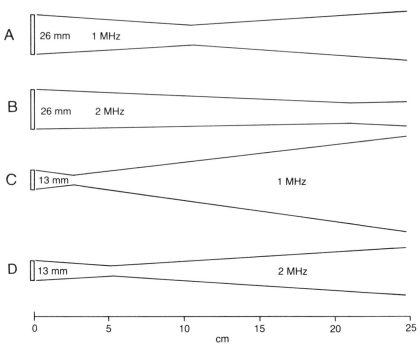

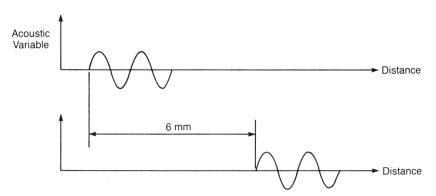

Figure 8.4. Figure for Exercise 8.78. (From Kremkau FW: Basic principles and biological effects of ultrasound. *In* Resnick MI, Sanders RC [eds]: Ultrasound in Urology. Baltimore, Williams & Wilkins, 1979. Reprinted with permission.)

Figure 8.5. Figure for Exercise 8.79. (From Kremkau FW: Basic principles and biological effects of ultrasound. *In* Resnick MI, Sanders RC [eds]: Ultrasound in Urology. Baltimore, Williams & Wilkins, 1979. Reprinted with permission.)

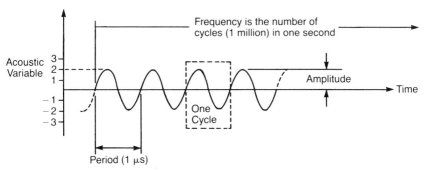

Figure 8.6. Figure for Exercise 8.80. (From Kremkau FW: Basic principles and biological effects of ultrasound. *In* Resnick MI, Sanders RC [eds]: Ultrasound in Urology. Baltimore, Williams & Wilkins, 1979. Reprinted with permission.)

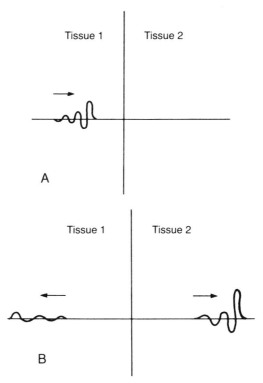

Figure 8.7. Figure for Exercise 8.81. (From Kremkau FW: Ultrasound instrumentation: physical principles. *In* Callen PW [ed]: Ultrasonography in Obstetrics and Gynecology. Philadelphia, WB Saunders, 1982. Reprinted with permission.)

8.80 In Figure 8.6, the frequency is _____ MHz, the period is _____ μs, the amplitude is _____ units, the wave type is (continuous-wave or pulsed), and for soft tissue the wavelength is _____ mm.

8.81 In Figure 8.7, which of the following have occurred?
 a. reflection
 b. refraction
 c. transmission
 d. a and b
 e. a and c

8.82 In Figure 8.8, which is the higher frequency pulse?
 a. a
 b. b
 c. neither

8.83 In Figure 8.8, which pulse travels faster?
 a. a
 b. b
 c. neither

8.84 In Figure 8.8, which pulse travels farther (experiences less attenuation)?
 a. a
 b. b
 c. neither

8.85 In Figure 8.8, which pulse has the better axial resolution?
 a. a
 b. b
 c. neither

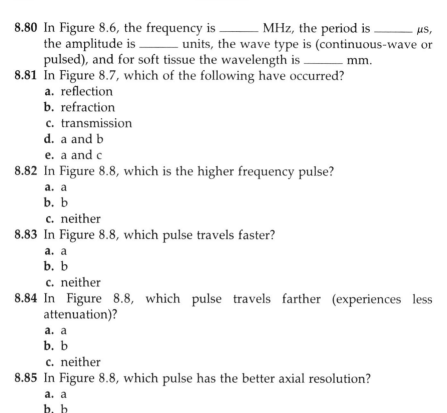

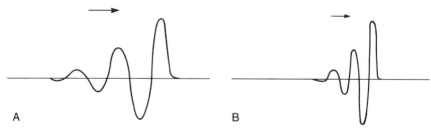

Figure 8.8. Figure for Exercises 8.82 to 8.86. (From Kremkau FW: Ultrasound instrumentation: physical principles. *In* Callen PW [ed]: Ultrasonography in Obstetrics and Gynecology. Philadelphia, WB Saunders, 1982. Reprinted with permission.)

8.86 In Figure 8.8, which pulse has the greater amplitude?
  a. a
  b. b
  c. neither

8.87 As frequency increases, which of the following (more than one) decrease?
  a. period
  b. wavelength
  c. propagation speed
  d. amplitude
  e. intensity
  f. attenuation coefficient
  g. half-intensity depth
  h. reflection coefficient
  i. transmission coefficient
  j. refraction
  k. pulse duration
  l. spatial pulse length
  m. pulse repetition frequency
  n. pulse repetition period
  o. duty factor
  p. near-zone length
  q. imaging depth
  r. axial resolution
  s. impedance

8.88 Fill in the missing values in the table.

Incident Frequency (MHz)	Flow Speed (cm/s)	Angle (°)	Reflected Frequency (MHz)	Doppler Shift (kHz)
2	30	0	(a)	(b)
4	30	0	(c)	(d)
8	30	0	(e)	(f)
2	50	(g)	2.0000	(h)
4	50	(i)	(j)	1.3
8	50	30	(k)	(l)

  a. _____   **d.** _____
  b. _____   **e.** _____
  c. _____   **f.** _____

g. ——   **j.** ——
h. ——   **k.** ——
i. ——   **l.** ——

8.89 Compensation makes up for the fact that echoes from deeper reflectors arrive weaker. True or false?

8.90 In which direction is blood flow in Figure 1.2 (p. 3)?

Glossary

Absorption. Conversion of sound to heat.

Acceleration. Change in velocity divided by time over which the change occurs.

Acoustic. Having to do with sound.

Acoustic propagation properties. Characteristics of a medium that affect the propagation of sound through it.

Acoustic variables. Pressure, density, temperature, and particle motion—things that are functions of space and time in a sound wave.

Aliasing. Improper doppler shift information from a pulsed doppler instrument when true doppler shift exceeds half the pulse repetition frequency.

Amplification. Increasing small voltages to larger ones.

Amplifier. A device that accomplishes amplification.

Amplitude. Maximum variation of an acoustic variable or voltage.

Analog. Related to a procedure or system in which data are represented by continuously variable physical quantities (e.g., electric voltage).

Anechoic. Having no echoes.

Annular array. Array made up of ring-shaped elements arranged concentrically.

221

Array. Transducer array.

Attenuation. Decrease in amplitude and intensity as a wave travels through a medium.

Attenuation coefficient. Attenuation per unit length of wave travel.

Autocorrelation. A rapid technique for obtaining mean doppler shift frequency. This technique is used in color-flow instruments.

Axial. In the direction of the transducer axis (sound-travel direction).

Axial resolution. Minimum reflector separation along the sound path required for separate reflections to be produced.

B mode. Mode of operation in which the display records a spot brightening for each echo pulse delivered from the receiver.

B scan. A brightness image that represents a cross section of the object through the scanning plane.

Backscatter. Sound scattered back in the direction from which it originally came.

Baseline shift. Movement of the zero doppler-shift frequency or zero flow speed line up or down on a spectral display.

Bandwidth. Range of frequencies contained in an ultrasound pulse or echo.

Beam area. Cross-sectional area of a sound beam.

Beam axis. A straight line down the center of a sound beam.

Bernoulli effect. Pressure reduction in a region of high-flow speed.

Bidirectional. Indicating doppler instruments capable of distinguishing between positive and negative doppler shifts (forward and reverse flow).

Bit. Binary digit.

Bruit. Audible sounds (using a stethoscope) originating in vessels with disturbed or turbulent flow.

Cathode ray tube. A display device that produces an image by scanning an electron beam over a phosphor-coated screen.

Cavitation (acoustic). Production and behavior of bubbles by sound.

Clutter. Noise in the doppler signal generally caused by high-amplitude, doppler-shifted echoes from heart or vessel walls.

Color flow. The presentation of two-dimensional, real-time doppler shift information superimposed on a real-time, gray-scale anatomic cross-sectional image. Flow directions toward and away from the transducer (i.e., positive and negative doppler shifts) are presented as different colors on the display.

Compensation. Equalizing received reflection amplitude differences caused by attenuation and differences in reflector depth.

Compliance. Distensibility. Nonrigid stretchability of vessels.

Continuous mode. Continuous-wave mode.

Continuous wave. A wave in which cycles repeat indefinitely; not pulsed.

Continuous wave doppler. A doppler device or procedure that uses continuous-wave ultrasound.

Continuous-wave mode. Mode of operation in which continuous-wave sound is used.

Contrast resolution. Ability of a gray-scale display to distinguish between echoes of slightly different amplitude or intensity.

cos. Abbreviation for cosine.

Cosine. The cosine of an angle in a right triangle is the length of the adjacent divided by the length of the hypotenuse (longest side).

Coupling medium. Oil or gel used to provide a good sound path between the transducer and the skin.

Critical reynolds number. Reynolds number above which turbulence occurs.

Cross talk. Leakage of strong signals in one direction channel of a doppler receiver into the other channel. Can produce the doppler mirror-image artifact.

cw. Abbreviation for continuous wave.

Cycle. Complete variation of an acoustic variable.

Damping. Material placed behind the rear face of a transducer element to reduce pulse duration; also, the process of pulse duration reduction.

dB. Abbreviation for decibel.

Dead zone. Region close to the transducer in which imaging cannot be performed.

Decibel. Unit of power or intensity ratio; the number of decibels is 10 times the logarithm (to the base 10) of the power or intensity ratio.

Density. Mass divided by volume.

Digital. Related to a procedure or system in which data are represented by discrete units (numerical digits).

Disc. Thin, flat circular object.

Displacement. Distance that an object has moved.

Disturbed flow. Flow that cannot be described by straight, parallel streamlines.

Doppler angle. The angle between the sound beam and the flow direction.

Doppler effect. Frequency change of reflected sound wave as a result of reflector motion relative to transducer.

Doppler equation. The mathematical description of the relationship between doppler shift, frequency, angle, propagation speed, and motion.

Doppler sample volume. See sample volume.

Doppler shift. Reflected frequency minus incident frequency. Change in frequency due to motion.

Doppler spectrum. The range of frequencies present in doppler-shifted echoes.

Duplex instrument. An ultrasound instrument that combines gray-scale sonography with pulsed doppler and possibly continuous-wave doppler.

Duty factor. Fraction of time that pulsed ultrasound is on. Sometimes called duty cycle.

Dynamic focusing. Continuously variable-received focus that follows the changing position of the transmitted pulse.

Dynamic imaging. Rapid-frame-sequence imaging.

Dynamic range. Ratio (in decibels) of largest power to smallest power that a system can handle or of the largest to the smallest intensity of a group of echoes.

Echo. Reflection.

Eddies. See vortices.

Electric current. The rate of flow of electrons in an electric conductor.

Electric pulse. A brief excursion of electric voltage from its normal value.

Electric resistance. The characteristic of electric components that limits the electric current for a given voltage.

Electric resistor. A device that limits the electric current for a given voltage.

Electric voltage. Electric potential or potential difference expressed in volts.

Electricity. A form of energy associated with the displacement or flow of electrons.

Energy. Capability of doing work.

Energy, kinetic. Energy of motion.

Energy, potential. Energy of position or state.

Enhancement. Increase in reflection amplitude from reflectors that lie behind a weakly attenuating structure.

Far zone. The region of a sound beam in which the beam diameter increases as the distance from the transducer increases.

Fast fourier transform (FFT). Digital computer implementation of the fourier transform.

Filter. An electrical circuit that passes frequencies within a certain range.

Flow rate. Volume flow.

Flow speed. Rate of motion of a portion of a flowing fluid.

Focal length. Distance from focused transducer to center of focal region or to the location of the spatial peak intensity.

Focal region. Region of minimum beam diameter and area.

Focus. To concentrate the sound beam into a smaller beam area than would exist otherwise.

Focusing, dynamic. See dynamic focusing.

Force. That which changes the state of rest or motion of an object.

Fourier analysis. The application of the fourier transform to determine the frequency components present.

Fourier transform. A mathematical technique for obtaining a doppler spectrum.

Frame. Single display image produced by one complete scan of the sound beam.

Frame rate. Number of frames displayed per unit time.

Frequency. Number of cycles per unit time.

Frequency, doppler shift. See doppler shift.

Frequency spectrum. The range of frequencies present. In a doppler instrument, the range of doppler shift frequencies present in the returning echoes.

Gain. Ratio of output to input electrical power.

Generator gate. The electronic portion of a pulsed doppler system that converts the continuous voltage of the voltage generator to a pulsed voltage.

Gray scale. Continuous range of brightnesses between white and black.

Gray-scale display. Display in which several values of spot brightness may be displayed.

Heat. Energy resulting from thermal molecular motion.

Hertz. Unit of frequency, one cycle per second; unit of pulse repetition frequency, one pulse per second.

Hydrophone. A small transducer element mounted on the end of a narrow tube.

Hyperechoic. Having relatively strong echoes.

Hypoechoic. Having relatively weak echoes.

Hz. Abbreviation for hertz.

Impedance (acoustic). Density multiplied by sound propagation speed.

Impedance (flow). Resistance to pulsatile flow. Pressure difference divided by flow rate.

Incidence angle. Angle between incident sound direction and line perpendicular to boundary of the medium.

Inertia. Resistance to acceleration.

Intensity. Power divided by area.

Internal focus. A focus produced by a curved transducer element.

kHz. Abbreviation for kilohertz.

Kilohertz. One thousand hertz.

Laminar flow. Flow in which fluid layers slide over each other to produce a parabolic flow speed profile.

Lateral. Perpendicular to the direction of sound travel.

Lateral resolution. Minimum reflector separation perpendicular to the sound path required for separate reflections to be produced.

Linear array. Array made up of rectangular elements in a line.

Linear-phased array. Linear array operated by applying voltage pulses to all elements but with small time differences.

Linear-switched array. Linear array operated by applying voltage pulses to groups of elements sequentially.

Longitudinal wave. Wave in which the particle motion is parallel to the direction of wave travel (compressional wave).

Mass. Measure of an object's resistance to acceleration.

Matching layer. Material placed in front of the front face of a transducer element to reduce the reflection at the transducer surface.

Medium. Material through which a wave travels.

Megahertz. One million hertz.

MHz. Abbreviation for megahertz.

Mirror-image artifact. In sonography, duplication of an object on the opposite side of a strong reflector. In doppler, duplication of the spectrum on the other side of the base line.

Multigate doppler. A pulsed doppler with more than one gate.

Multiple reflection. Several reflections produced by a pulse encountering a pair of reflectors (reverberation).

Near zone. The region of a sound beam in which the beam diameter decreases as the distance from the transducer increases.

Noise. Unwanted acoustic or electric signals.

Nyquist limit. The doppler shift above which aliasing occurs (half the pulse-repetition frequency).

Oblique incidence. Sound direction is not perpendicular to media boundary.

Operating frequency. Preferred frequency of operation of a transducer.

Parabolic flow. Laminar flow.

Particle. Small portion of a medium.

Particle motion. Displacement, speed, velocity, and acceleration of a particle.

Perpendicular. Geometrically related by 90 degrees.

Perpendicular incidence. Sound direction is perpendicular to media boundary.

Phantom. Tissue-equivalent materials that have some characteristics representative of tissues (e.g., scattering or attenuation properties).

Phase quadrature. Two signals differing by one fourth of a cycle.

Piezoelectricity. Conversion of pressure to electric voltage.

Pixel. Picture element; the unit into which imaging and doppler information is divided for storage and display in a digital instrument.

Plug flow. Flow with all fluid portions traveling with nearly the same flow speed and direction.

Poise. Unit of viscosity.

Poiseuille's law. The mathematical description of the dependence of flow rate on pressure, vessel length and radius, and fluid viscosity.

Power. Rate at which work is done; rate at which energy is transferred.

Pressure. Force divided by area.

PRF. Abbreviation for pulse repetition frequency.

Probe. Transducer assembly.

Propagation. Progression or travel.

Propagation speed. Speed with which a wave moves through a medium.

Pulsatility index. A description of the relationship between peak systolic and end diastolic flow speeds or doppler shifts.

Pulse. A brief excursion of a quantity from its normal value; a few cycles.

Pulse duration. Time from beginning to end of a pulse.

Pulse-echo diagnostic ultrasound. Ultrasound imaging and flow measurement in which pulses are reflected and used to produce a display.

Pulse repetition frequency. Number of pulses per unit time. Sometimes called pulse repetition rate.

Pulsed doppler. A doppler device or procedure that uses pulsed-wave ultrasound.

Pulsed mode. Mode of operation in which pulsed ultrasound is used.

Pulsed ultrasound. Ultrasound produced in pulse form by applying electric pulses or voltages of a few cycles to the transducer.

Range ambiguity. Incorrect range determination for echoes caused by a pulse repetition frequency that is too high.

Range gating. Selecting depth from which echoes are accepted based on echo arrival time.

Rayl. Unit of acoustic impedance.

Rayleigh scattering. Scattering of sound by particles that are small compared to wavelength.

Real-time. Imaging with a rapid-frame-sequence display.

Real-time display. A display that continuously images moving structures or changing scan planes.

Receiver gate. A device that allows only echoes from a selected depth (arrival time) to pass.

Reflection. Portion of sound returned from a boundary of a medium (echo).

Reflection angle. Angle between reflected sound direction and a line perpendicular to the boundary of a medium.

Reflection, specular. See specular reflection.

Reflector. Medium boundary that produces a reflection; reflecting surface.

Refraction. Change of sound direction on passing from one medium to another.

Reject. Elimination of voltages below a set level (called the threshold or rejection level).

Resistance (flow). Pressure difference divided by flow rate for steady flow.

Resonance frequency. Operating frequency.

Reverberation. Multiple reflections.

Reynolds number. A number that depends on flow speed and viscosity and predicts the onset of turbulence.

Sample volume. The region from which doppler shifts are acquired.

Scan converter. A device that stores imaging information in one scanning format and reads it out for display in another.

Scan line. A line produced on a display by moving a spot (produced by an electron beam) across the display face at constant speed. An echo line written into memory.

Scanning. Sweeping a sound beam to produce an image.

Scatterer. An object that scatters sound because of its small size or its surface roughness.

Scattering. Diffusion or redirection of sound in several directions on encountering a particle suspension or a rough surface.

Sensitivity. Ability of an imaging system to detect weak reflections.

Shadowing. Reduction in reflection amplitude from reflectors that lie behind a strongly reflecting or attenuating structure.

Signal. Information-bearing voltages in an electrical circuit. An acoustic, visual, electrical, or other conveyance of information.

Sound. Traveling wave of acoustic variables.

Sound beam. The region of a medium that contains virtually all the sound produced by a transducer.

Source. An emitter of ultrasound (transducer).

Spatial pulse length. Length of space over which a pulse occurs.

Speckle. The granular appearance of images or doppler spectra caused by the interference of echoes from the distribution of scatterers in tissue.

Spectral analysis. Separating frequencies in a doppler signal for display as a doppler spectrum.

Spectral broadening. The widening of the doppler shift spectrum, i.e., the increase of the range of doppler shift frequencies present, owing to a broader range of flow speeds encountered by the sound beam. This occurs for normal flow in smaller vessels and for turbulent flow in any vessel.

Spectral display. Visual display of a doppler spectrum.

Spectral width. Range of doppler shifts or flow speeds present at a given point in time.

Spectrum. Range of frequencies.

Spectrum analyzer. A device that derives a frequency spectrum from a complex signal.

Specular reflection. Reflection from a smooth boundary.

Speed. Displacement divided by time over which displacement occurs.

Stenosis. Narrowing of a vessel.

Stoke. Unit of kinematic viscosity.

Streamline. A line representing the path of motion of a particle of fluid.

Strength. Nonspecific term referring to amplitude or intensity.

Temperature. Condition of a body that determines transfer of heat to or from other bodies.

Test object. A device designed to measure some characteristic of an imaging system without having tissue-like properties.

TGC. Compensation; time gain compensation.

Threshold. See reject.

Transducer. Device that converts energy from one form to another.

Transducer array. Transducer assembly containing more than one transducer element.

Transducer assembly. Transducer element with damping and matching materials assembled in a case.

Transducer element. Piece of piezoelectric material in a transducer assembly.

Transmission angle. Angle between transmitted sound direction and a line perpendicular to the boundary of a medium.

Turbulence. Random, chaotic, multidirectional flow of a fluid.

Turbulent flow. See turbulence.

Ultrasound. Sound of frequency greater than 20 kHz.

Ultrasound transducer. Device that converts electric energy to ultrasound energy and vice versa.

Variable focusing. Transmit focus with various focal lengths.

Vector. A quantity with magnitude and direction.

Velocity. Speed with direction of motion specified.

Viscosity. Resistance of a fluid to flow.

Viscosity, kinematic. Viscosity divided by density.

Voltage pulse. Brief excursion of voltage from its normal value.

Volume flow. Volume of fluid passing a point per unit time (second or minute).

Vortices. Regions of circular flow patterns. Present in turbulence.

Wall filter. An electrical filter that passes frequencies above a set level and eliminates strong low-frequency doppler shifts from pulsating heart or vessel walls.

Wave. Traveling variation of wave variables.

Wave variables. Things that are functions of space and time in a wave.

Wave velocity. See propagation speed.

Wavelength. Length of space over which a cycle occurs.

Window. An anechoic region underneath a region of echo frequencies presented on a doppler spectral display.

Work. Force multiplied by displacement.

Wrap around. The shift of doppler information on a spectral display to the wrong side of the base line (caused by aliasing).

Zero-crossing counter. A simple analog detector that yields mean doppler shift as a function of time.

Zero shift. See baseline shift.

Answers to Exercises in the Text

Chapter 1

1.1   d, e
1.2   motion
1.3   a, b, e
1.4   blood, loudspeaker, display
1.5   angle

Chapter 2

2.1   pulses, ultrasound, echoes, image
2.2   pulse, echo
2.3   strength (intensity, amplitude)
2.4   parallel
2.5   origin (starting point)
2.6   rectangular
2.7   pie-slice
2.8   pulse, echo, location, strength, location, brightness
2.9   a
2.10 a. 4; b. 1; c. 3; d. 5; e. 2
2.11 propagation speeds, equal
2.12 d
2.13 e

2.14   impedances
2.15   false
2.16   a. 4; b. 3; c. 2; d. 1
2.17   a, d
2.18   c
2.19   focal
2.20   true
2.21   false
2.22   a
2.23   e
2.24   resolution, imaging depth
2.25   2, 10
2.26   b
2.27   d
2.28   d
2.29   b
2.30   b
2.31   d
2.32   reflections or echoes
2.33   strength, direction, time
2.34   display, voltages
2.35   receiver
2.36   pulser
2.37   receiver
2.38   a
2.39   f
2.40   b
2.41   a
2.42   false
2.43   mechanical, electronic
2.44   frame
2.45   pulsed
2.46   false (latter portion)
2.47   increase
2.48   improved, decreases, increased
2.49   freeze, frame
2.50 $\frac{1000}{20}$ = 50 lines per frame (one scan line for each pulse)
2.51   c, d, e
2.52   a. 1; b. 2; c. 2
2.53   separation
2.54   weaker
2.55   b
2.56   true
2.57   refraction (double image)

Chapter 3

3.1   a, c, d, e, g, h
3.2   capillaries
3.3   a, b, f
3.4   d
3.5   c
3.6   stream
3.7   plasma, erythrocytes, water
3.8   d
3.9   a
3.10   e
3.11   b
3.12   c
3.13   viscosity
3.14   kinematic viscosity
3.15   density
3.16   1.05 g/mL, 0.035 poise, 0.033 stoke
3.17   force
3.18   c
3.19   difference, gradient
3.20   a
3.21   pump, gravity
3.22   difference, distance or separation
3.23   pressure, resistance
3.24   d
3.25   decreases
3.26   d
3.27   c
3.28   vessels
3.29   e
3.30   d
3.31   d
3.32   b
3.33   b
3.34   d
3.35   e
3.36   e
3.37   e
3.38   b or c
3.39   disturbed
3.40   turbulent
3.41   reynolds

3.42 stenosis
3.43 d
3.44 a
3.45 decrease
3.46 increase
3.47 e
3.48 a
3.49 a
3.50 e
3.51 33 cm/s
3.52 16 cm/s, 960; 64 cm/s, 1920; 16 cm/s, 960
3.53 d
3.54 e

Chapter 4

4.1   doppler, flow
4.2   frequency or wavelength
4.3   frequency or wavelength, motion
4.4   higher
4.5   lower
4.6   equal to
4.7   motion
4.8   0.02, 1.02
4.9   0.026
4.10 −0.026
4.11 reflected, incident
4.12 cosine
4.13 0.01, 1.01 (the doppler shift is cut in half)
4.14 0, 1.00 (no doppler shift at 90 degrees)
4.15 110
4.16 a. 1.62; b. 0; c. 50; d. 2.5; e. 6.49; f. 0; g. 150; h. 5; i. 14.6; j. 2.81;
      k. 60; l. 90; m. 100; n. 3.25; o. 100; p. 30; q. 5; r. 0
4.17 c
4.18 0.26 kHz
4.19 0.44
4.20 1.95
4.21 100 cm/s
4.22 50 cm/s
4.23 decrease
4.24 increases
4.25 5 MHz

4.26 -5 MHz
4.27 0 MHz
4.28 infinity (shock wave)
4.29 2.5 MHz
4.30 false
4.31 at the blood vessel wall boundary
4.32 yes. Without them the doppler shifted sound would not be reflected back to the transducer.
4.33 b
4.34 c
4.35 doppler angle
4.36 speed, angle
4.37 a
4.38 doubled
4.39 doubled
4.40 decreased
4.41 a. 325 kHz; b. 347 kHz; c. 694 kHz
4.42 3.85 MHz, 7.70 MHz
4.43 96 cm/s, 192 cm/s
4.44 7.7 MHz
4.45 154 cm/s
4.46 5, 0.1
4.47 θ_1, θ_2, no, θ_3, θ_1 and θ_3, 90 degrees
4.48 b
4.49 d
4.50 low
4.51 100
4.52 100
4.53 two
4.54 It decreases because doppler angle is increasing.

Chapter 5

5.1 false
5.2 direction, bidirectional
5.3 false
5.4 voltage generator, source transducer, receiving transducer, receiver, loudspeaker, memory, display
5.5 amplitude, frequency
5.6 frequency, time
5.7 gray, color
5.8 flow velocities

5.9   true
5.10 gates, transducers
5.11 continuous, pulsed
5.12 depths, arrival time
5.13 false
5.14 profile
5.15 true
5.16 e
5.17 gates
5.18 flow, anatomy
5.19 d
5.20 red, blue, blue, red
5.21 fast fourier transform
5.22 autocorrelation, mean
5.23 b
5.24 FFT
5.25 no
5.26 pulsed
5.27 a. pulsed; b. pulsed; c. continuous (no gate)
5.28 50 seconds
5.29 100 seconds
5.30 damped, longer, efficient
5.31 c
5.32 c
5.33 e
5.34 b
5.35 continuous-wave, pulsed-wave, duplex, color-flow
5.36 continuous-wave
5.37 pulsed-wave
5.38 duplex
5.39 color-flow
5.40 receiver
5.41 a
5.42 doppler angle
5.43 cathode, ray
5.44 wall, wall, thump
5.45 5, 30, gate, pulse
5.46 nyquist
5.47 range ambiguity
5.48 continuous wave
5.49 false
5.50 false
5.51 mechanical scanner

5.52   false
5.53   c
5.54   b
5.55   c
5.56   e
5.57   e
5.58   false
5.59   false (e.g., Color Plate VIII)

Chapter 6

6.1   components or frequencies, order
6.2   c
6.3   a
6.4   shifts
6.5   speeds, directions
6.6   single
6.7   a
6.8   e
6.9   amplitude, power, time
6.10   second
6.11   brightness, gray, scale
6.12   d
6.13   a
6.14   c
6.15   b
6.16   d
6.17   true
6.18   false
6.19   laminar
6.20   b
6.21   e (a, c, or d)
6.22   false
6.23   e
6.24   a
6.25   a
6.26   c
6.27   false
6.28   false
6.29   e (b, c, d)
6.30   false
6.31   b

6.32   c
6.33   a
6.34   a. 2; b. 1; c. 3
6.35   narrow
6.36   higher
6.37   false
6.38   false (Fig. 6.16)
6.39   c
6.40   true
6.41   varies, compliant, higher, lower
6.42   small doppler angle
6.43   large doppler angle
6.44   false
6.45   false
6.46   e

Chapter 7

7.1   a
7.2   e (a, b, d)
7.3   d
7.4   b
7.5   b
7.6   b
7.7   c
7.8   d
7.9   e
7.10   b
7.11   e
7.12   b
7.13   e
7.14   c
7.15   yes—less attenuation, greater penetration, later echoes
7.16   yes—doppler shift increases with increasing frequency
7.17   d
7.18   a
7.19   e (c and d)
7.20   e
7.21   a. 3; b. 4; c. 3; d. 2; e. 1
7.22   b, c, d
7.23   liquid, string
7.24   rods, water, alcohol

7.25   a. 1; b. 2; c. 3; d. 6; e. 4; f. 3; g. 7; h. 7
7.26   a. 4; b. 4; c. 3; d. 2; e. 1; f. 1; g. 1
7.27   true
7.28   true
7.29   1
7.30   distance
7.31   distances or depths
7.32   tissues
7.33   false
7.34   d
7.35   false
7.36   b
7.37   d
7.38   b, c, d, e
7.39   true
7.40   transducer
7.41   true
7.42   b
7.43   a
7.44   a
7.45   b
7.46   e
7.47   false
7.48   d
7.49   a. 2; b. 1, 2; c. 2, 3
7.50   a. 2; b. 3; c. 1
7.51   false
7.52   false
7.53   b
7.54   no
7.55   yes
7.56   b and d
7.57   c
7.58   c
7.59   e
7.60   e
7.61   e
7.62   a
7.63   d
7.64   b
7.65   d
7.66   e
7.67   c, d, e

7.68   b
7.69   a, b, d
7.70   e
7.71   b
7.72   a

Chapter 8

8.1   doppler shift
8.2   false
8.3   one, two
8.4   frequencies
8.5   false
8.6   speed
8.7   gate
8.8   display
8.9   gate, voltage generator
8.10   depth
8.11   true
8.12   false
8.13   true
8.14   2.6
8.15   true
8.16   continuous wave
8.17   b
8.18   a
8.19   c
8.20   d
8.21   e
8.22   e
8.23   a
8.24   a
8.25   c
8.26   c
8.27   false (only true near the transducer)
8.28   false (only true for normal incidence or oblique incidence when densities and propagation speeds of the media are equal)
8.29   false (see comment for 8.28)
8.30   c
8.31   d
8.32   d
8.33   false (6 bits)

8.34 d
8.35 a
8.36 b
8.37 c
8.38 d (areas are 284 and 3 mm^2)
8.39 c
8.40 d
8.41 e
8.42 c
8.43 a
8.44 a
8.45 a
8.46 d (b and c)
8.47 c
8.48 c
8.49 e (d and a or b)
8.50 c
8.51 false
8.52 b
8.53 c
8.54 See page 245.
8.55 See page 246.
8.56 See page 246.
8.57 See page 247.
8.58 See page 247.
8.59 e
8.60 a
8.61 b
8.62 d
8.63 b
8.64 a, b, c, d, e
8.65 c
8.66 e
8.67 a
8.68 e (a, b, c)
8.69 d
8.70 b
8.71 a
8.72 false
8.73 false
8.74 e
8.75 b
8.76 a. 2; b. 2; c. 1.5 mm; d. 3 mm; e. 10 μs; f. 100 kHz; g. 2 μs; h. 1 μs; i. 1 MHz; j. 0.2; k. 1.5 mm/μs

8.77 c, a, b, b

8.78 longer, longer, none; b; a, b, and d

8.79 pulsed, 1.5, 1.5, 3

8.80 1, 1, 2, continuous-wave, 1.54

8.81 e

8.82 b

8.83 c

8.84 a

8.85 b

8.86 c

8.87 a, b, g, k, l, o, q, r

8.88 a. 2.0008; b. 0.8; c. 2.0016; d. 1.6; e. 2.0031; f. 3.1; g. 90; h. 0.0; i. 60; j. 4.0013; k. 8.0046; l. 4.6

8.89 true

8.90 right to left (above base line but note "inverted")

8.54

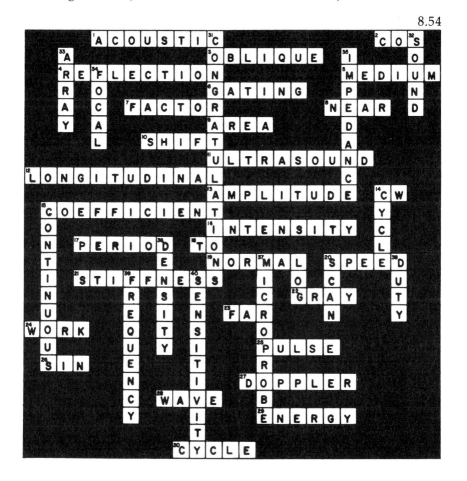

8.55

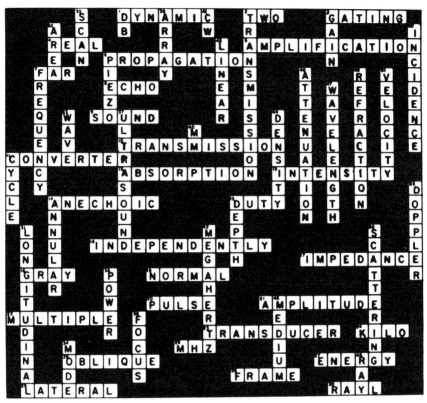

8.56

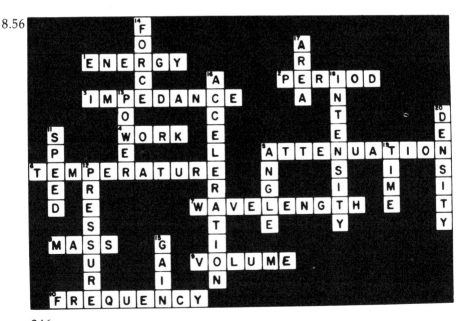

8.57 **START**

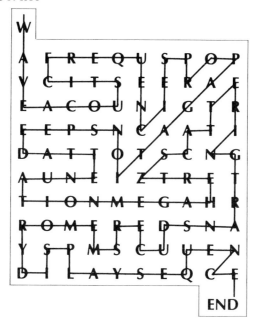

8.58

```
. . . E . . . . . . . . U . . . .
. . . . V . . . . . . L D . . . .
. . C . . A . . . . . T O . . . .
. . O . . . W . . . R P . . . . . T
. . L . . . . - . A P . . . . . F .
. . O . . . . . S L . . . . . I . .
. . R . . . . O E U . . . . H . . .
. . - . . . U R . . O . . S . . . E
. . F . . N - . . . . Y U - . . . V .
. . L . D A . . . C . R N . . A . .
. . O A N . . . N . E . . I W . . .
. . W G L . . E . L . . . - T . . .
. . L . . I U . P . . . D . . N . .
. E . . . Q A P . . . E . . . . O .
. . . . . E . O S . . S . . . . . C
. . . R . D . . I L . . . . . . . .
. . F . . . . . U N . . . . . . . .
. . . . . . . P . . G . . . . . . .
```

Appendix A
Symbols and Abbreviations

a	attenuation
A	beam area, tube or vessel cross-sectional area
c	sound propagation speed
cos	cosine
d	vessel diameter
d_m	maximum unambiguous imaging or doppler sample depth
f	frequency, source frequency
f_D	doppler shift
f_e	emitted frequency
f_o	source or operating frequency, emitted frequency
f_r	received frequency
I	intensity
L	vessel or tube length, sound path length
n	number of cycles in a pulse
P	power, pressure
Q	volume flow
r	vessel radius
R	flow resistance
Re	reynolds number
SPL	spatial pulse length
v	reflector or scatterer speed, flow speed
v_a	average flow speed

v_m maximum flow speed
v_r receiver speed
v_s source speed
λ wavelength
λ_e emitted wavelength
λ_o source wavelength
ρ density
θ doppler angle
θ_D doppler angle
θ_i incidence angle
θ_r reflection angle
θ_t transmission angle
ν viscosity

Appendix B
Comprehensive Examination

This examination should take less than 2 hours to complete (averaging less than 1 minute per question). The answers are found on pages 270 to 274.

1. In general, as a reflector approaches a transducer at constant speed, the doppler-shift frequency
   a. increases
   b. decreases
   c. remains constant
   d. b or c
   e. none of the above
2. A reduction in diameter produces a(n)
   a. increase in flow resistance
   b. decrease in area
   c. increase in flow speed
   d. decrease in flow speed
   e. all of the above
3. Which of the following increases vascular flow resistance?
   a. decreasing vessel length
   b. decreasing viscosity
   c. decreasing vessel diameter
   d. decreasing pressure
   e. decreasing flow speed

4. Which of the following frequencies is in the ultrasound range?
   a. 15 Hz
   b. 15 kHz
   c. 15 MHz
   d. 17,000 Hz
   e. 17 km

5. The average propagation speed in soft tissues is
   a. 1.54 mm/μs
   b. 0.501 m/s
   c. 1540 dB/cm
   d. 37.0 km/min
   e. 1–10 MHz

6. The propagation speed in blood is
   a. 0.330 mm/μs
   b. 1.54 mm/μs
   c. 1.57 mm/μs
   d. 1.75 mm/μs
   e. none of the above

7. The doppler effect occurs as
   a. the leukocytes move through the plasma
   b. the erythrocytes move through the plasma
   c. the erythrocytes move through the serum
   d. blood moves relative to the vessel wall
   e. all of the above

8. When a reflector is moving toward the transducer
   a. propagation velocity increases
   b. propagation velocity decreases
   c. doppler shift is positive (frequency increases)
   d. doppler shift is negative (frequency decreases)
   e. none of the above

9. Doppler sample volume is determined by
   a. beam width
   b. pulse length
   c. frequency
   d. receiver gate length
   e. all of the above

10. Doppler shift frequencies
    a. are generally in the audible range
    b. are usually above 1 MHz
    c. can be applied to a loudspeaker
    d. a and b
    e. a and c

11. Spatial pulse length equals the number of cycles in the pulse times
    a. period
    b. impedance
    c. beam width
    d. resolution
    e. wavelength
12. Which of the following has a significant dependence on frequency in soft tissues?
    a. propagation speed
    b. density
    c. stiffness
    d. attenuation
    e. impedance
13. The attenuation of 5 MHz ultrasound in 2 cm of soft tissue is
    a. 5 dB/cm
    b. 5 dB
    c. 2.5 MHz/cm
    d. 2 cm
    e. 5 dB/MHz
14. Impedance equals propagation speed times
    a. density
    b. stiffness
    c. frequency
    d. attenuation
    e. path length
15. For perpendicular incidence, if the intensity transmission coefficient is 96 percent, what is the intensity reflection coefficient?
    a. 2 percent
    b. 4 percent
    c. 6 percent
    d. 8 percent
    e. 10 percent
16. The quantitative presentation of frequencies contained in echoes is called
    a. preamplification
    b. digitizing
    c. optical encoding
    d. spectral analysis
    e. all of the above
17. The range equation describes the relationship of
    a. reflector distance, propagation time, and sound speed
    b. distance, propagation time, and reflection coefficient

c. number of cows and sheep on a ranch

d. propagation time, sound speed, and transducer frequency

e. dynamic range and system sensitivity

18. Axial resolution in a system equals

    a. four times the spatial pulse length

    b. ratio of reflector size to transducer frequency

    c. maximum reflector separation expected to be displayed

    d. minimum reflector separation expected to be displayed

    e. spatial pulse length

19. The doppler frequency shift is caused by

    a. relative motion between the transducer and the reflector

    b. patient shivering in a cool room

    c. a high transducer frequency and real-time scanner

    d. small reflectors in the transducer beam

    e. changing transducer thickness

20. A small (relative to the transducer wavelength) reflector is said to _____ an incident sound beam.

    a. focus

    b. speculate

    c. scatter

    d. shatter

    e. amplify

21. The frequency of an ultrasound transducer is primarily determined by which of the following:

    a. element diameter

    b. element thickness

    c. speed of sound in tissue

    d. voltage applied

    e. all of the above

22. The fundamental operating principle of medical ultrasound transducers is

    a. Snell's law

    b. Doppler's law

    c. magnetostrictive effect

    d. piezoelectric effect

    e. impedance effect

23. The axial resolution of a transducer is primarily determined by

    a. spatial pulse length

    b. the near-field limit

    c. the transducer diameter

    d. the acoustic impedance of tissue

    e. density

24. The lateral resolution of a transducer is primarily determined by
    a. spatial pulse length
    b. the near-field limit
    c. the transducer diameter
    d. the acoustic impedance of tissue
    e. applied voltage

25. Which of the following quantities varies most with distance from the transducer face?
    a. axial resolution
    b. lateral resolution
    c. frequency
    d. wavelength
    e. period

26. If the near-zone length of an unfocused transducer 13 mm in diameter extends (in soft tissue) 6 cm from the transducer face, at which of the following distances from the face can the lateral resolution be improved by focusing the sound from this transducer?
    a. 13 cm
    b. 8 cm
    c. 3 cm
    d. 9 cm
    e. none of the above

27. The lateral resolution of an ultrasound *system* depends upon
    a. the transducer diameter
    b. the transducer frequency
    c. the speed of sound in soft tissue
    d. memory and display
    e. all of the above

28. Which of the following is a characteristic of a medium through which sound is propagating?
    a. impedance
    b. intensity
    c. amplitude
    d. frequency
    e. period

29. For perpendicular incidence, if the impedances of the two media are the same, there will be no
    a. inflation
    b. reflection
    c. refraction
    d. calibration
    e. b and c

30. Increasing frequency
    a. improves resolution
    b. increases half-intensity depth
    c. increases refraction
    d. a and b
    e. a and c
31. Increasing intensity produced by the transducer
    a. is accomplished by increasing pulser voltage
    b. increases sensitivity of the system
    c. increases probability of biologic effects
    d. all of the above
    e. none of the above
32. Ultrasound bioeffects
    a. do not occur
    b. do not occur with diagnostic instruments
    c. are not confirmed below 100 mW/cm^2 SPTA
    d. b and c
    e. none of the above
33. Diagnostic ultrasound frequency range is
    a. 2 to 10 mHz
    b. 2 to 10 kHz
    c. 2 to 10 MHz
    d. 3 to 15 kHz
    e. none of the above
34. If propagation speeds of two media are equal, incidence angle equals
    a. reflection angle
    b. transmission angle
    c. doppler angle
    d. a and b
    e. b and c
35. What is the wavelength of 1 MHz ultrasound in tissue with a propagation speed 1540 m/s?
    a. 1×10^6 m
    b. 1.54 mm
    c. 1540 m
    d. 1.54 cm
    e. 0.77 cm
36. The doppler effect is a change in
    a. intensity
    b. wavelength
    c. frequency
    d. all of the above
    e. b and c

37. What determines the lower and upper limits of frequency range useful in diagnostic ultrasound?
    a. resolution and imaging depth
    b. intensity and resolution
    c. intensity and propagation speed
    d. scattering and impedance
    e. impedance and wavelength
38. If no refraction occurs as an oblique sound beam passes through the boundary between two materials, what is unchanged as the boundary is crossed?
    a. impedance
    b. propagation speed
    c. intensity
    d. sound direction
    e. b and d
39. Attenuation along a sound path is a decrease in
    a. frequency
    b. amplitude
    c. intensity
    d. b and c
    e. impedance
40. Reverberation causes us to think there are reflectors that are too great in
    a. impedance
    b. attenuation
    c. range
    d. size
    e. number
41. Doppler shift is zero when the angle between the sound direction and the movement (flow) direction is _____ degrees.
    a. 30
    b. 60
    c. 90
    d. 45
    e. none of the above
42. An important factor in the selection of a transducer for a specific application is the ultrasonic attenuation of tissue. Due to this attenuation, a 7.5 MHz transducer should generally be used for
    a. imaging deep structures
    b. imaging shallow structures
    c. imaging both deep and shallow structures
    d. imaging adult intracranial structures
    e. all of the above

43. A real-time scan
  a. consists of many frames produced per second
  b. depends on how short a time the sonographer takes to make a scan
  c. is made only between 8 A.M. and 5 P.M.
  d. gives a gray-scale image, whereas other scans give only an M-mode display
  e. none of the above

44. The standard U.S. television scanning format has _____ lines per frame and _____ frames per second.
  a. 625, 25
  b. 512, 512
  c. 512, 640
  d. 525, 30
  e. 625, 30

45. In an ultrasound imaging instrument, a cathode ray tube is used as a
  a. pulser
  b. receiver
  c. memory
  d. display
  e. scan convector

46. The dynamic range of an ultrasound system is defined as
  a. the speed with which ultrasound examination can be performed
  b. the range over which the transducer can be manipulated
  c. the ratio of the maximum to the minimum intensity that can be displayed
  d. the range of pulser voltages applied to the transducer
  e. none of the above

47. The compensation (swept gain, etc.) control serves to
  a. compensate for machine instability in the warm-up time
  b. compensate for attenuation
  c. compensate for transducer aging and the ambient light in the examining area
  d. decrease patient examination time
  e. none of the above

48. A digital scan converter is a
  a. compressor
  b. receiver
  c. display
  d. computer memory
  e. none of the above

49. Mechanical real-time devices may be designed such that
  a. a transducer is "rocked" at the skin surface
  b. a transducer is not moved at all

c. a transducer is rocked and the beam passed through a liquid path
d. a and c
e. all of the above

50. Phased array systems involve the sequential switching of a small group of elements along the array.
a. true
b. false

51. Duplex doppler presents
a. anatomic (structural) data
b. physiologic (flow) data
c. impedance data
d. more than one of the above
e. all of the above

52. Doppler shift frequencies are usually in a relatively narrow range above 20 kHz.
a. true
b. false

53. Enhancement is caused by
a. strongly reflecting structure
b. weakly attenuating structure
c. strongly attenuating structure
d. frequency error
e. propagation speed error

54. Postprocessing is the process of assigning numbers to be placed in memory.
a. true
b. false

55. In a digital instrument, echo intensity is represented in memory by
a. positive charge distribution
b. a number
c. electron density of the scan converter writing beam
d. a and c
e. all of the above

56. Increasing the gain generally produces the same effect as
a. decreasing the attenuation
b. increasing the compression
c. increasing the rectification
d. both b and c
e. all of the above

57. A gray-scale display shows
a. gray color on a white background
b. reflections with one brightness level

   c. a white color on a gray background
   d. a range of reflection amplitudes or intensities
   e. none of the above
58. Which of the following is performed in an imaging receiver?
   a. amplification
   b. compensation
   c. compression
   d. demodulation
   e. all of the above
59. Continuous-wave sound is used in
   a. all ultrasound imaging instruments
   b. only bistable instruments
   c. all doppler instruments
   d. some doppler instruments
   e. some M-Mode instruments
60. Increasing the pulse repetition frequency
   a. improves resolution
   b. increases maximum unambiguous depth
   c. decreases maximum unambiguous depth
   d. both a and b
   e. both a and c
61. If four shades of gray are shown on a display, each twice the brightness of the next brightest one, the brightest shade is _____ times the brightness of the dimmest shade.
   a. 2
   b. 4
   c. 8
   d. 16
   e. 32
62. The dynamic range displayed in Exercise 61 is _____ dB.
   a. 100
   b. 9
   c. 5
   d. 2
   e. 0
63. The 100-mm test object measures
   a. resolution
   b. pulse duration
   c. SATA intensity
   d. wavelength
   e. all of the above

64. The following measure acoustic output:
    a. hydrophone
    b. optical encoder
    c. 100-mm test object
    d. all of the above
    e. none of the above·
65. Real-time imaging is made possible by
    a. scan converters
    b. mechanically driven transducers
    c. gray-scale display
    d. arrays
    e. both b and d
66. Gain and attenuation are usually given in
    a. dB
    b. dB/cm
    c. cm
    d. cm/dB
    e. none of the above
67. Gray-scale display is made possible by
    a. array transducers
    b. cathode-ray storage tubes
    c. scan converters
    d. b and c
    e. all of the above
68. An advantage of cw doppler over pulsed doppler is
    a. depth information
    b. bidirectional
    c. no aliasing
    d. b and c
    e. all of the above
69. In doppler color-flow instruments, color represents
    a. sign (+ or −) of doppler shift
    b. flow direction
    c. magnitude of the doppler shift
    d. amplitude of the doppler shift
    e. a and b
70. Attenuation is corrected for by
    a. demodulation
    b. desegregation
    c. decompression
    d. compensation
    e. remuneration

71. What must be known in order to calculate distance to a reflector?
    a. attenuation, speed, density
    b. attenuation, impedance
    c. attenuation, absorption
    d. travel time, speed
    e. density, speed

72. Which of the following improve sound transmission from the transducer element into the tissue?
    a. matching layer
    b. doppler effect
    c. damping material
    d. coupling medium
    e. a and d

73. Lateral resolution is improved by
    a. damping
    b. pulsing
    c. focusing
    d. reflecting
    e. absorbing

74. The doppler effect for a scatterer moving toward the sound source causes the scattered sound (compared to incident sound) received by the transducer to have
    a. increased intensity
    b. decreased intensity
    c. increased impedance
    d. increased frequency
    e. decreased impedance

75. Axial resolution is improved by
    a. damping
    b. pulsing
    c. focusing
    d. reflecting
    e. absorbing

76. Duplex doppler instruments include _____.
    a. pulsed doppler
    b. cw doppler
    c. B-scan imaging
    d. dynamic imaging
    e. more than one of the above

77. If the doppler shifts from normal and stenotic arteries are 4 kHz and 10 kHz, respectively, for which will there be a problem (aliasing) with a pulse repetition frequency of 7 kHz?

    a. normal
    b. stenotic
    c. both
    d. neither

78. The receiver in a doppler system compares the _____ of the voltage generator and the echo voltage from the transducer.
    a. wavelength
    b. intensity
    c. impedance
    d. frequency
    e. all of the above

79. A digital imaging instrument divides the cross-sectional image into _____.
    a. frequencies
    b. bits
    c. pixels
    d. binaries
    e. wavelengths

80. Which of the following produce(s) a sector-scan format?
    a. rotating mechanical real-time transducer
    b. oscillating mechanical real-time transducer
    c. phased array
    d. oscillating mirror
    e. all of the above

81. The piezoelectric effect describes how _____ is converted into _____ by a _____.
    a. electricity, an image, display
    b. incident sound, reflected sound, boundary
    c. ultrasound, electricity, transducer
    d. ultrasound, heat, tissue
    e. none of the above

82. Propagation speed in soft tissues
    a. is directly proportional to frequency
    b. is inversely proportional to frequency
    c. is directly proportional to intensity
    d. is inversely proportional to intensity
    e. none of the above

83. The frequencies used in diagnostic ultrasound imaging
    a. are much lower than those used in doppler measurements
    b. determine imaging depth in tissue
    c. determine imaging resolution
    d. all of the above
    e. b and c

84. As frequency is increased
    a. wavelength increases
    b. a three-cycle ultrasound pulse decreases in length
    c. imaging depth decreases
    d. propagation velocity decreases
    e. b and c

85. In the Doppler equation

$$f_D = \frac{2\,fv}{c - v}$$

which can normally be ignored?
    a. v in the denominator
    b. v in the numerator
    c. f
    d. f_D
    e. b and c

86. For which of the following is the reflected frequency less than the incident frequency?
    a. advancing flow
    b. receding flow
    c. perpendicular flow
    d. laminar flow
    e. all of the above

87. Focusing
    a. improves lateral resolution
    b. improves axial resolution
    c. increases beam width in the focal region
    d. shortens pulse length
    e. increases duty factor

88. Doppler ultrasound can measure flow in
    a. heart
    b. veins
    c. arterioles
    d. capillaries
    e. a and b

89. Which of the following are fluids?
    a. gas
    b. liquid
    c. solid
    d. a and b
    e. all of the above

90. The mass per unit volume of a fluid is called its
    a. resistance
    b. viscosity
    c. kinematic viscosity
    d. impedance
    e. density

91. The resistance to flow offered by a fluid is called
    a. resistance
    b. viscosity
    c. kinematic viscosity
    d. impedance
    e. density

92. Viscosity divided by density is called
    a. resistance
    b. viscosity
    c. kinematic viscosity
    d. impedance
    e. density

93. If the following is increased, flow increases.
    a. pressure difference
    b. pressure gradient
    c. resistance
    d. a and b
    e. all of the above

94. Flow resistance depends most strongly on which of the following?
    a. vessel length
    b. vessel radius
    c. blood viscosity
    d. all of the above
    e. none of the above

95. Proximal to, at, and distal to a stenosis _____ must be constant.
    a. laminar flow
    b. disturbed flow
    c. turbulent flow
    d. volume flow
    e. none of the above

96. Added forward flow and flow reversal in diastole are results of _____ flow.
    a. volume
    b. turbulence
    c. laminar

    d. disturbed

    e. pulsatile

97. Turbulence generally occurs when reynolds number exceeds

    a. 100

    b. 200

    c. 1000

    d. 2000

    e. a and b

98. As stenosis diameter decreases, the following pass through a maximum:

    a. flow speed at the stenosis

    b. flow speed proximal to stenosis

    c. volume flow

    d. doppler shift at the stenosis

    e. a and d

99. Which has the highest speed of sound?

    a. air

    b. water

    c. lung

    d. soft tissue

    e. bone

100. The highest number that an 8-bit memory can store is

    a. 31

    b. 64

    c. 127

    d. 255

    e. 256

101. The doppler shift (kHz) for 4 MHz, 50 cm/s, and 60 degrees is

    a. 0.5

    b. 1.0

    c. 1.3

    d. 2.6

    e. 5.0

102. Physiologic flow speeds can be as much as _____ percent of the propagation speed in soft tissues.

    a. 0.01

    b. 0.3

    c. 5

    d. 10

    e. 50

103. Which doppler angle gives the greatest doppler shift?

    a. −90

    b. −45

c. 0

d. 45

e. 90

104. Doppler shift frequency is not dependent on
   a. amplitude
   b. flow speed
   c. operating frequency
   d. doppler angle
   e. propagation speed

105. The fourier-transform technique is not used in color-flow instruments because it is not _____ enough.
   a. slow
   b. fast
   c. bright
   d. cheap
   e. none of the above

106. Which of the following on a color-flow display is (are) presented in real-time?
   a. gray-scale anatomy
   b. flow direction
   c. doppler spectrum
   d. a and b
   e. all of the above

107. For a 5-MHz instrument and 60-degree doppler angle, a 100-Hz filter eliminates flow speeds below
   a. 1 cm/s
   b. 2 cm/s
   c. 3 cm/s
   d. 4 cm/s
   e. 5 cm/s

108. For a 7.5-MHz instrument and 0-degree doppler angle, a 100-Hz filter eliminates flow speeds below
   a. 1 cm/s
   b. 2 cm/s
   c. 3 cm/s
   d. 4 cm/s
   e. 5 cm/s

109. The functions of a doppler receiver include which of the following?
   a. amplification
   b. phase-quadrature detection
   c. demodulation
   d. reject
   e. all of the above

110. A later receiver gate time means a _____ sample volume depth.
    a. earlier
    b. shallower
    c. deeper
    d. stronger
    e. none of the above
111. The doppler shift is typically _____ of the source frequency.
    a. 1/1000th
    b. 1/100th
    c. 1/10th
    d. 10 times
    e. 100 times
112. Approximately _____ pulses are required to obtain one line of color-flow information.
    a. 1
    b. 10
    c. 100
    d. 1000
    e. 1,000,000
113. There are approximately _____ samples per line on a color-flow display.
    a. 2
    b. 20
    c. 200
    d. 2000
    e. 2,000,000
114. Which of the following instruments can produce aliasing?
    a. continuous-wave doppler
    b. pulsed doppler
    c. duplex
    d. color flow
    e. more than one of the above
115. For normal flow in a large vessel, particularly in systole, a _____ range of doppler-shift frequencies is received.
    a. narrow
    b. broad
    c. steady
    d. disturbed
    e. all of the above
116. Doppler signal power is proportional to
    a. volume flow
    b. flow speed

    c. doppler angle

    d. cell density

    e. more than one of the above

117. Stenosis affects

    a. peak systolic flow speed

    b. end diastolic flow speed

    c. spectral broadening

    d. window

    e. all of the above

118. Spectral broadening is a _____ of the spectral trace.

    a. vertical thickening

    b. horizontal thickening

    c. brightening

    d. darkening

    e. horizontal shift

119. As stenosis is increased, which of the following increase(s)?

    a. vessel diameter

    b. systolic doppler shift

    c. diastolic doppler shift

    d. spectral broadening

    e. more than one of the above

120. Flow reversal in diastole indicates

    a. stenosis

    b. aneurysm

    c. high distal impedance

    d. low distal impedance

    e. more than one of the above

Comprehensive Exam Answers

Following each answer is the section number in which the subject is discussed. Most answers also have explanatory comments.

1. d. 4.1, 4.3. If the transducer is in the path of the reflector, answer c) is correct because doppler angle is zero. If this is not the case, then b) is correct because the doppler angle will increase (decreasing the doppler shift) as the reflector approaches.
2. e. 3.2, 3.3. The diameter referred to can be either the total vessel diameter or the diameter of a small portion of it (stenosis). For the former, d) is correct. For the latter, c) is correct. In either case, a) and b) are correct.
3. c. 3.2. Poiseuille's equation shows that resistance increases with increasing vessel length, increasing fluid viscosity, or decreasing vessel diameter.
4. c. 2.1. Ultrasound is sound of frequency greater than 20 kHz (0.02 MHz). Answer e) is not in frequency units.
5. a. 2.1. Propagation speeds in soft tissues are in the range of about 1.4 to 1.6 mm/μs. Answers c) and e) are not in speed units.
6. c. 4.1. Slightly higher than for soft tissues.
7. d. 4.1. The blood cells move along with the plasma, not through it.
8. c. 2.1, 4.1. Propagation speed is determined by the medium, not by motion.
9. e. 5.2.
10. e. 4.1.

11. e. 2.1. The wavelength is the length of each cycle in a pulse.

12. d. 2.1. Propagation speed and impedance increase only slightly with frequency.

13. b. 2.1. The attenuation coefficient of 5-MHz ultrasound is approximately 2.5 dB/cm. The attenuation coefficient times the path length yields the attenuation in dB. Only answer b) is given in attenuation (dB) units.

14. a. 2.1. This is the characteristic impedance.

15. b. 2.1. If 96 percent of the intensity is transmitted, 4 percent was reflected. (What is not reflected is transmitted, i.e., the two must add up to 100 percent.)

16. d. 5.1 and 6.1. Spectral comes from "spectrum," referring to color spectrum. A prism is an optical spectrum analyzer that breaks down white light into its component colors.

17. a. 2.1. Reflector distance equals ½ × speed × time.

18. d. 2.2. If reflectors are separated by less than the axial resolution, they are not separated on the display.

19. a. 4.1.

20. c. 2.1. Scattering occurs with rough surfaces and with heterogeneous media (made up of small particles relative to the wavelength). Large, flat surfaces produce specular reflections.

21. b. 2.2 The operating frequency of a transducer is such that its thickness is equal to one half the wavelength in the transducer element material.

22. d. 2.2. Transducer elements expand and contract when a voltage is applied, and, conversely, when returning echoes apply pressure to the element, a voltage is generated.

23. a. 2.2. Axial resolution is equal to one half spatial pulse length.

24. c. 2.2. Lateral resolution is equal to beam width. Near-zone length is dependent on transducer diameter and, thus, so is the lateral resolution at any given distance from the transducer.

25. b. 2.2. Beam width changes with distance from transducer and, thus, also lateral resolution.

26. c. 2.2. Focusing can only be accomplished in the near zone of a beam.

27. e. 2.2. Answers a, b, and c all affect the beam. Resolution of the system is also affected by the display and the electronics of the instrument.

28. a. 2.1. All the others are characteristics of the sound.

29. e. 2.1. For perpendicular incidence, there is no refraction. For equal impedances, there is no reflection.

30. a. 2.1, 2.2. Half-intensity depth decreases with increasing frequency and frequency has no effect on refraction.

31. d. 2.3 and 7.3.

32. c. 7.3. This is the AIUM statement on in vivo mammalian bioeffects.

33. c. 2.1, 2.2. Frequencies lower than this range do not provide the needed resolution whereas frequencies greater than this range do not allow for adequate imaging depth for medical purposes.

34. d. 2.1. Incidence angle always equals reflection angle and, for equal propagation speeds, equals transmission angle as well.

35. b. 2.1. Wavelength is equal to propagation speed divided by frequency.

36. e. 4.1. If frequency changes, wavelength changes also.

37. a. 2.1, 2.2. See answer to question 33.

38. e. 2.1. No refraction means that there is no change in sound direction. This is a result of no change in propagation speed (equal propagation speeds on both sides of the boundary).

39. d. 2.1.

40. e. 2.4. Reverberation adds additional reflectors on the display deeper than the true ones.

41. c. 4.3.

42. b. 2.1. A 7.5-MHz transducer can image to only a few centimeters in tissue.

43. a. 2.2 and 2.3. The other answers make little sense.

44. d. 2.3.

45. d. 2.3.

46. c. 2.3.

47. b. 2.3.

48. d. 2.3.

49. e. 2.2. In the answer b), the beam can be reflected off an oscillating acoustic mirror (reflector).

50. b. 2.2. This is a description of a linear switched or sequenced array rather than a phased array.

51. d. 5.3. Answers a) and b) are both correct. Anatomic data are provided by the real-time B scan, and physiologic data are provided by the pulsed doppler portion of the instrument.

52. b. 4.1. Physiologic doppler shift frequencies are usually in the audible frequency range.

53. b. 2.4.

54. b. 2.3. Postprocessing is the assignment of display brightness to numbers coming out of memory.

55. b. 2.3.

56. a. 2.1 and 2.3. Increasing gain and decreasing attenuation each increase echo intensity.

57. d. 2.3.

58. e. 2.3.

59. d. 5.1. All imaging instruments and some doppler instruments use pulsed ultrasound.

60. c. 7.1. Pulse repetition frequency has no effect on resolution.

61. c. 2.3.

62. b. 2.3. A factor of 8 is three doublings, i.e., 3 plus 3 plus 3 dB.

63. a. 7.2.

64. a. 7.2.

65. e. 2.2.

66. a. 2.1 and 2.3.

67. c. 2.3.

68. c. 5.1 and 5.2.

69. e. 5.4.

70. d. 2.3.

71. d. 2.1. Distance equals one half speed times round-trip time.

72. e. 2.2. The matching layer improves sound transmission by reducing the reflection at the transducer-skin boundary. A coupling medium improves it by removing the air layer between the transducer and the skin.

73. c. 2.2.

74. d. 4.1.

75. a. 2.2.

76. e. 5.3. They include pulsed doppler (and sometimes continuous doppler) and dynamic imaging.

77. c. 7.1. Both doppler shifts exceed one half the pulse repetition frequency. The problem will be aliasing.

78. d. 5.1.

79. c. 2.3.

80. e. 2.2.

81. c. 2.2.

82. e. 2.1. Propagation speed is independent of frequency and intensity.

83. e. 2.1 and 2.2.

84. e. 2.1.

85. a. 4.1. Because physiologic speeds (v) are small compared to the speed of sound (c) in tissues.

86. b. 4.1.

87. a. 2.2.

88. e. 3.1. Arterioles and capillaries are too small.

89. d. 3.1.

90. e. 3.1.

91. b. 3.1.

92. c. 3.1.

93. d. 3.2. This is Poiseuille's law. Increasing resistance *decreases* flow.

94. b. 3.2. It depends on radius to the fourth power.
95. d. 3.3. This is the continuity rule.
96. e. 3.4. Also results of distensible vessels.
97. d. 3.2.
98. e. 3.3. See Figure 3.9.
99. e. 2.1. Because it is a solid.
100. d. 2.3. Therefore, it can display 256 shades (0–255).
101. c. 4.1. Assuming a *reflector* moving at 50 cm/s.
102. b. 4.2. That is, about 5 m/s.
103. c. 4.3. Smaller angle, larger cosine, larger shift.
104. a. 4.1.
105. b. 5.4. Thus, autocorrelation is commonly used.
106. d. 5.4. The spectrum can be shown *in addition* to the color-flow display.
107. c. 4.1. $v = \dfrac{77 \times 0.100}{5 \times 0.5} = 3.08$
108. b. 4.1. $v = \dfrac{77 \times 0.100}{7.5 \times 0.5} = 2.05$
109. e. 5.1.
110. c. 5.2. 13 microseconds of delay per centimeter of depth.
111. a. 4.1. Because flow speeds are typically 1/1000th the speed of sound in tissues.
112. b. 5.4. The range is about 4 to 32.
113. c. 5.4. The range is about 40 to 400.
114. e. 7.1. Any pulsed instrument (b, c, d) can.
115. a. 3.2. This is called plug flow.
116. d. 5.1.
117. e. 3.3. A stenosis generally increases a), b), and c) and decreases d).
118. a. 6.3. That is, a widening of the spectrum.
119. e. 3.3, 6.3. b, c, d, (a) is *decreased*.
120. c. 6.3. The blood flows back out of the high impedance vascular bed during the low-pressure portion of the cardiac cycle.

References

1. Strandness DE: Vascular testing, a new turf battle? Admin Radiol, September, p. 30, 1987.
2. Eden A: The beginnings of doppler. *In* Aaslid R (ed): Transcranial Doppler Sonography. New York, Springer-Verlag, 1986, pp. 1–9.
3. Eden A: Johann Christian Doppler. Ultrasound Med Biol *11*:L537–L539, 1985.
4. White DN: Johann Christian Doppler and his effect—a brief history. Ultrasound Med Biol *8*:583–591, 1982.
5. Jonkman EJ: Doppler research in the nineteenth century. Ultrasound Med Biol *6*:1–5, 1980.
6. Weld PW: History of doppler echocardiography. J Cardiovasc Ultrasonography *7*:285–292, 1988.
7. Patterson EC: Why the doppler effect? Am Scientist *76*:533, 1988.
8. Kremkau FW: Diagnostic Ultrasound: Principles, Instruments, and Exercises, 3rd edition. Philadelphia, WB Saunders, 1989.
9. Trahey GE, Hubbard SM, von Ramm OT: Angle independent ultrasonic blood flow detection by frame-to-frame correlation of B-mode images. Ultrasonics *26*:271–276, 1988.
10. Embree PM, O'Brien Jr, WD: The accurate ultrasonic measurement of volume flow of blood by time domain correlation. Proc IEEE Ultrasonics Symp., pp. 963–966, 1985.
11. Evans DH, McDicken WN, Skidmore R, Woodcock JP: Doppler Ultrasound: Physics, Instrumentation, and Clinical Applications. New York, Wiley & Sons, 1989.

12. Atkinson P, Woodcock JP: Doppler Ultrasound and Its Use in Clinical Measurement. New York, Academic Press, 1982.
13. Taylor KJW, Burns PN, Wells PNT (eds): Clinical Applications of Doppler Ultrasound. New York, Raven Press, 1988.
14. Jaffe CC (ed): Clinics in Diagnostic Ultrasound. Vol. 13: Vascular and Doppler Ultrasound. New York, Churchill Livingstone, 1984.
15. Hershey FB, Barnes RW, Sumner DS: Noninvasive Diagnosis of Vascular Disease. Pasadena, Appleton-Davies, 1984.
16. Nanda NC: Doppler Echocardiography. New York, Igaku-Shoin, 1985.
17. Hatle L, Angelsen B: Doppler Ultrasound in Cardiology: Physical Principles and Clinical Applications. Philadelphia, Lea & Febiger, 1985.
18. Kisslo J, Adams D, Mark DB (eds): Clinics in Diagnostic Ultrasound, Vol. 17: Basic Doppler Echocardiography. New York, Churchill Livingstone, 1986.
19. Zweibel WJ (ed): Introduction to Vascular Ultrasonography. Orlando, Grune & Stratton, 1986.
20. Maulik D, McNellis D (eds): Doppler Ultrasound Measurement of Maternal-Fetal Hemodynamics. Ithaca, Perinatology Press, 1987.
21. Grant EG, White EM (eds): Duplex Sonography. New York, Springer-Verlag, 1988.
22. Aaslid R (ed): Transcranial Doppler Sonography. New York, Springer-Verlag, 1986.
23. Kremkau FW, Taylor KJW: Artifacts in ultrasound imaging. J Ultrasound Med 5:227–237, 1986.
24. Guyton AC: Textbook of Medical Physiology, 7th edition. Philadelphia, WB Saunders Company, 1986.
25. Milnor WR: Hemodynamics, 2nd edition. Baltimore, Williams & Wilkins, 1989.
26. Fung YC: Biodynamics of Circulation. New York, Springer-Verlag, 1984.
27. Noordergraaf A: Circulatory System Dynamics. New York, Academic Press, 1978.
28. McDonald DA: Blood Flow in Arteries. London, Edward Arnold, 1960.
29. Spencer MP, Reid JM: Quantitation of carotid stenosis with continuous wave (CW) doppler ultrasound. Stroke 10(3):326–330, 1979.
30. Bradley EL, Sacerio J: The velocity of ultrasound in human blood under varying physiologic parameters. J Surg Res 12:290–297,1972.
31. Goss SA, Johnston RL, Dunn F: Comprehensive compilation of empirical ultrasonic properties of mammalian tissues. J Acoust Soc Am 64(2), 1978.

32. Censor D: Acoustical doppler effect analysis—is it a valid method? J Acoust Soc Am *83*(4), 1988.

33. Wells PNT, Luckman NP, Skidmore R: A second order approximation in the doppler equation. Ultrasound Med Biol *15*:73–75, 1989.

34. Kremkau FW: Source of doppler shift in blood flow. Ultrasound Med Biol., in press.

35. Fuss EL: The technology of burglar alarm systems. Am Scientist *72*:334–337, 1984.

36. Luckman NP, Evans JM, Skidmore R, et al: Backscattered power in doppler signals. Ultrasound Med Biol *13*:L669–L670, 1987.

37. Beach KW, Lawrence R, Phillips DJ, et al: The systolic velocity criterion for diagnosing significant internal carotid artery stenoses. J Vascular Technol *13*:65–68, 1989.

38. Ku DN, Giddens DP, Phillips DJ, Strandness DE: Hemodynamics of the normal human carotid bifurcation: in vitro and in vivo studies. Ultrasound Med Biol *11*:13–26, 1985.

39. Phillips DJ, Beach KW, Primozich J, Strandness DE: Should results of ultrasound doppler studies be reported in units of frequency or velocity? Ultrasound Med Biol *15*:205–212, 1989.

40. Kremkau FW: Doppler shift frequency data. J Ultrasound Med *6*:167,1987.

41. Bracewell RN: The fourier transform. Scientific American *260*:86–95, 1989.

42. Gill RW: Measurement of blood flow by ultrasound: accuracy and sources of error. Ultrasound Med Biol *11*:625–641, 1985.

43. Kremkau FW: Letter to the editor. Ultrasound Med Biol *12*:L647, 1986.

44. Takeuchi Y: Color coded doppler scans. Ultrasound Med Biol *13*:L151, 1987.

45. Kremkau FW: Colour coded doppler scans. Ultrasound Med Biol *13*:L152, 1987.

46. White DN: Colour coded doppler systems. Ultrasound Med Biol *13*:L209, 1987.

47. Takeuchi H: Letter to the editor. Ultrasound Med Biol *13*:L210, 1987.

48. Burns PN: The physical principles of doppler and spectral analysis. J Clin Ultrasound *15*:567–590, 1987.

49. Roederer GO, Langlois YE, Chan AW, et al.: Ultrasonic duplex scanning of extracranial carotid arteries: improved accuracy using new features from the common carotid artery. J Cardiovasc Ultrasonography *1*:373–380, 1982.

50. Roederer GP, Langlois YE, Jager KA, et al: A simple spectral parameter for accurate classification of severe carotid disease. Bruit *8*:174–178, 1984.

51. Bluth EI, Stavros AT, Marich KW, et al: Carotid duplex sonography: a multicenter recommendation for standardized imaging and doppler criteria. RadioGraphics 8:487–506, 1988.

52. Taylor DC, Strandness DE: Carotid artery duplex scanning. J Clin Ultrasound 15:635–644, 1987.

53. Taylor KJW, Holland S: State-of-the-art doppler ultrasound I. Basic principles, instrumentation and pitfalls. Radiology 174:297–307.

54. Bom K, de Boo J, Rijsterborgh H: On the aliasing problem in pulsed doppler cardiac studies. J Clin Ultrasound 12:559–567, 1984.

55. Goldstein A: Range ambiguities in real-time ultrasound. J Clin Ultrasound 9:83, 1981.

56. Jawad IA, Taylor ML, Hudson FP, Sohn YH: Range ambiguity in pulsed doppler ultrasound: the ambiguity clarified? J Clin Ultrasound 13:475–479, 1985.

57. Gill RW, Kossoff MB, Kossoff G, Griffiths KA: New class of pulsed doppler vs ambiguity at short ranges. Radiology 173:272, 1989.

58. Boote EJ, Zagzebski JA: Performance tests of doppler ultrasound equipment with a tissue and blood-mimicking phantom. J Ultrasound Med 7:137–147, 1988.

59. Walker AR, Phillips DJ, Powers JE: Evaluating doppler devices using a string target. J Clin Ultrasound 10:25, 1982.

60. Goldstein A: Quality Assurance in Diagnostic Ultrasound. Bethesda, MD, American Institute of Ultrasound in Medicine, 1980.

61. Banjavic RA: Design and maintenance of a quality assurance program for diagnostic ultrasound equipment. Semin Ultrasound 4:10–26, 1983.

62. Williams AR: Ultrasound: Biological Effects and Potential Hazards. London, Academic Press, 1983.

63. NCRP: Biological Effects of Ultrasound: Mechanisms and Clinical Implications, NCRP Report No. 74. Bethesda, National Council on Radiation Protection and Measurements, NCRP Publications, 1983.

64. Nyborg WL: Ziskin MC (eds): Biological Effects of Ultrasound. New York, Churchill Livingstone, 1985.

65. AIUM: Safety Considerations for Diagnostic Ultrasound. Bethesda, American Institute of Ultrasound in Medicine, 1984.

66. Wells PNT (ed): The Safety of Diagnostic Ultrasound. London, British Institute of Radiology, 1987.

67. AIUM: Bioeffects considerations for the safety of diagnostic ultrasound. J Ultrasound Med 7(9):Supplement, 1988.

68. Kremkau FW: How safe is obstetric ultrasound? Contemporary OB/GYN 20:182–186, 1982.

69. Kremkau FW: Biological effects and possible hazards. Clin Obst Gynecol 10:395–405, 1983.

70. Kremkau FW: Safety and long-term effects of ultrasound: what to tell your patients. Clin Obstet Gynecol 27:269–275, 1984.

71. Kremkau FW: Biological effects and safety. *In* Sarti DA (ed): Diagnostic Ultrasound: Text and Cases, 2nd edition. Chicago, Year Book Medical Publishers, 1987, pp. 25–29.

72. Barnett SB, Kossoff G: Ultrasonic exposure in static and real time echography. Ultrasound Med Biol 8:273, 1982.

73. Carson PL, Fischella PR, Oughton TV: Ultrasonic power and intensities produced by diagnostic ultrasound equipment. Ultrasound Med Biol 3:341, 1978.

74. World Health Organization: Environmental Health Criteria 22-Ultrasound, 1982, p. 65.

75. Nyborg WL: Appendix: ultrasonic intensities generated by real-time devices, Chapter 2. *In* Winsberg F, Cooperberg PL (eds): Real-Time Ultrasonography Instrumentation (Clinics in Diagnostic Ultrasound 10), New York, Churchill Livingstone, 1982.

76. AIUM/NEMA: Appendix B: survey of exposure levels from current diagnostic ultrasound systems. J Ultrasound Med (suppl) 2:S31, 1983.

77. National Council on Radiation Protection and Measurements. NCRP Report, Biological Effects of Ultrasound: Mechanisms and Clinical Applications. No. 74, pp. 64–69, Bethesda, 1983.

78. AIUM: Acoustical Data for Diagnostic Ultrasound Equipment. Manufacturer's Commendation Panel, 1985.

79. Nyborg WL: Appendix: exposure parameters for diagnostic equipment, Chapter 14. *In* Nyborg WL, Ziskin MC (eds): Biological Effects of Ultrasound (Clinics in Diagnostic Ultrasound 16). New York: Churchill Livingstone, 1985.

80. Duck FA, Starritt HC, Aindow JD, et al: The output of pulse-echo ultrasound equipment: a survey of powers, pressures and intensities. Br J Radiol 58:989, 1985.

81. The Institute of Physical Sciences in Medicine: Physics in Medical Ultrasound, J.A. Evans (Ed.), Chapters 5–7, London, 1986.

82. Duck FA: The measurement of exposure to ultrasound and its application to estimates of ultrasound "dose." Phys Med Biol 32:316,1987.

83. Kremkau FW: Bioeffects and safety. *In* Chervenak F, Isaacson G, and Campbell S (eds): Textbook of Ultrasound in Obstetrics and Gynecology. Boston, Little, Brown, in press.

84. Smith SW, Stewart HF, Jenkins DP: A plane layered model to estimate in situ ultrasound exposures. Ultrasonics 23:31, 1985.

85. NCRP: Biological Effects of Ultrasound: Mechanisms and Clinical Implications. Report No. 74, pp. 37–39, Bethesda, National Council on Radiation Protection and Measurements, 1983.

86. Duck FA: Output data from European studies. Ultrasound Med Biol 15 (Supp 1): 61–64, 1989.

87. Ziskin MC, Petitti DB: Epidemiology of human exposure to ultrasound: a critical review. Ultrasound Med Biol 14:91–96, 1988.

88. Lyons EA, Dyke D, Toms M, Cheang M: In utero exposure to diagnostic ultrasound: a 6-year follow-up. Radiology 166:687–690, 1988.

89. Taylor KJW: A prudent approach to doppler ultrasound. Radiology 165:283–284, 1987.

90. Taylor KJW, Kremkau FW: Diminishing exposure to doppler ultrasound. J Diag Med Sonography 4:5–8, 1988.

Index

Page numbers in italics indicate illustrations; page numbers followed by (t) indicate tables.

281